DO
THIS
FOR
YOU

DO THIS FOR YOU

HOW TO BE A STRONG WOMAN FROM THE INSIDE OUT

KRISSY CELA

hachette
BOOKS

New York

Hachette Go, an imprint of Hachette Books
Hachette Book Group
1290 Avenue of the Americas
New York, NY 10104
HachetteGo.com
Facebook.com/HachetteGo
Instagram.com/HachetteGo

First Edition: January 2021

Hachette Books is a division of Hachette Book Group, Inc.
The Hachette Go and Hachette Books name and logos are trademarks
of Hachette Book Group, Inc.

The publisher is not responsible for websites (or their content) that are
not owned by the publisher.

Library of Congress Cataloging-in-Publication Data has been applied
for.

ISBNs: 978-0-306-92507-8 (trade paperback); 978-0-306-92508-5 (ebook)

Library of Congress Control Number: 2020948342

Printed in the United States of America

LSC-C

Printing 1, 2020

For the Tone & Sculpt community—my familia, always.

This is for you.

CONTENTS

Introduction 1

1. Find Your "Why" 5
2. Lose the Excuses 17
3. Maximize Your Time 35
4. Form Healthy Habits 43
5. Shift Your Perspective 61
6. Believe You Can 77
7. Find Your Tribe 85
8. Embrace the Fear 97
9. Be More Than Motivated 109
10. Build Your Strength 123
11. Love Your Food 147
12. Do This for You 177

Frequently Asked Questions 191
Your Action Plan 205
Acknowledgments 209
Notes 213

INTRODUCTION

When I was a little girl, my parents brought our family to England in search of a better life for their children. I didn't know how to speak English, I didn't understand British culture, and my family and I spent several years finding our feet. I was always taught that hard work and focus was all I needed to be successful. I worked hard at school, I focused, and it got me to university to study law. While there I discovered fitness. In the midst of heartbreak, moving away from my family and working three jobs (all before the age of twenty), I found my way into the gym. I was overwhelmed, stressed and almost ready to give in, when I found myself facing the leg press machine about to learn something new. I discovered healthy habits, strength and discipline. I found a routine. I started my Instagram page to keep me accountable and, before I knew it, I was part of a community of people who are now the most wonderful part of my journey: my Tone & Sculpt familia. Fitness, exercise and healthy eating saved me and made me my best self—and I'm determined to make you feel your best self through it too.

Whatever you've felt when it comes to exercise, what-ever you have experienced—the barriers, the hurdles, the obstacles—trust me, I've been there, I get it and I know how to overcome it. I am just like you. If you think I am superwoman or have some kind of magic energy, you're wrong. Fitness has not come naturally to me; I don't believe it comes naturally to anyone. Even the greatest sportswomen will tell you they may have a knack for a particular sport, but it is hard work, practice and determination that makes them great. It makes them the very best versions of themselves and the best in their sport as well. I have good days, great days and awful days too, but I'm here to teach you that, with the right mindset, you just keep going. The fact that you've picked up this book today is the start of your best fitness journey yet.

If anyone ever tells you their fitness journey was easy or that it all came together how they wanted it to, that it all happened with a smile on their face and a spring in their step, they're lying. Mine didn't. It took me a long time to finally find fitness and only when I was at a pretty low ebb did I realize what it could give me and how it could change my life.

Once I found it, it took a long time to switch my mindset from focusing on a physical aesthetic—a curvier physique in my case—to one that would see fitness for what it could give me for my whole life, not just for a few weeks or months. It took me months to properly form the habits that I want for you. I skipped workouts, restricted my diet and found it hard to make my health a habit. Working out and staying healthy is tough—if it was easy, everyone would do it and stick with it. It takes dedication, discipline and hardwired habits.

In this book, I will ask you to change some habits you've probably had for a pretty long time. I will ask you to completely reevaluate everything you've felt and thought so far about fitness and food and their roles in your life. I want you to stop seeing improvements as short-term changes or fixes and see them as lifelong habits. It's all in your grasp and while it might take a while to set those patterns, it's worth it in time. Habits don't change overnight, but they stay with you forever once they're formed. You learned the habit of brushing your teeth as a toddler. Now try to imagine your life without a toothbrush... You're probably cringing at the thought of it!

If you form positive habits, hardwire them and reverse some of your thinking about food, you'll live a longer, happier and healthier life. There won't be extreme fluctuations, highs or lows; there won't be unhealthy eating habits with your diet and food intake constantly changing. Instead, there'll be consistency, knowledge and an understanding of how to mindfully manage your fitness and eating habits for the rest of your life. Imagine a life where it's second for you to work out and make the right choices without feeling you're depriving yourself. Imagine feeling sated, well rested, strong, healthy, happy and fresh—all of this is possible with time, discipline and a willingness to change.

Of course, there will be times when the going gets tough. You won't finish every session on a high; you'll have times when you feel ragged, when it's all you can do to get to the end of the workout in one piece. There'll be times when you'll be breathing so heavily and feel so exhausted that you'll struggle to lift your arms to drive home or to make your dinner. But I want you to get comfortable with being uncomfortable. Some workouts will go your way and they'll feel like second nature, some won't. Changing your fitness levels is tough. Getting better isn't easy. You're going to break yourself down to rebuild yourself back up again and that's going to come with some discomfort. You're going to ache as you'll be using muscles you haven't used in a really long time. You might question why you're doing it because it's hard. You might even feel ready to quit. That's when I need you to embrace the discomfort, the breathlessness, the feeling that you can't do one more rep. You can and you will if you lean in and just keep going.

I want this book to be your action plan. It won't give you a quick fix or a fitness plan that promises you a perfect body (whatever that is) in a few weeks, or even a few months...if any book promises to do that, don't buy it! This book is to get you thinking about your well-being, because that is your priority. Until I can get you believing *that*, your fitness will just remain something you remember on occasion. By the end of this book, you will be ready to make fitness and healthy living second nature and as normal for you as getting dressed. Yes, there may be days when you stay in your pajamas, lie in bed late or feel like watching the TV all day, but even on those days, you will rely on yourself to move, to work out and to do something for you.

Throughout the book you'll find tasks designed to get you thinking about your health and healthy habits. I want you to answer each task honestly, spend time with the book and know that we all start somewhere. Being fit and healthy is possible for all of us. There is no perfect design or one-size-fits-all model. Everyone's fitness journey is unique and designed just for them. The only person you are in competition with is yourself. No one else matters. The whole point of fitness for me (and now for you) is to use the time, effort and routine to focus on yourself and your well-being. That's all.

I just want this book to be right for you. I've poured my heart into it to give you all the information and guidance you need to kick-start your fitness journey and make better changes in your life—because you matter.

CHAPTER 1

FIND YOUR "WHY"

First, I just want to say well done and thank you so much for picking up this book! You have made an important decision to work on yourself and your fitness and well-being. You probably have a really good reason for reading this and I am here to help you at every step. This journey is ongoing and now that you're part of my familia, I'm with you for life!

Every journey needs to start with a purpose. Whether it's fitness, nutrition or even starting college or university, you have to have a reason why you're starting that journey, why it's important to you and why you're going to keep showing up and making progress. Think about it: when we go to college or university, it's usually because we enjoy a particular subject and we want to learn more; we want to get a job in a certain field or we are preparing for another training course or experience. Your fitness journey will be short-lived unless you define your reasons for it. Of course, you are training to keep fit and healthy, that's the general reason why all of us should do some form of exercise. But, to keep going, to keep you on the path of fitness, you need to refine that reason.

An author and speaker who I find inspiring is Simon Sinek. He talks a lot about the word "why." An expert in leadership, he writes that leaders, whatever field they're in, need to start with the question, "why?" They need to focus on *why* they are doing something, rather than *what* they are doing, in order to truly influence and inspire people. Now, I'm not about to teach you all about leadership—that's Simon's job—but what I am here to tell you is that you are the leader of your life and your greatest "why" is your health and happiness. It sounds scary and it requires you to be open to change and a challenge, but the rewards are endless.

When I first read Simon's book *Start with Why*, I thought about my own fitness journey and how I'd got here.[1] Fitness came to me at a time when my life was very unsettled and it took me a while to figure out my "why." I'd spent a few years on what felt like a conveyor belt. I was in a relationship that was no good for me, I was lacking in confidence, I was no longer living with my family, I wasn't even living in a fixed place and I was working a few jobs to make ends meet while trying to put myself through university. It was really hard. There were so many times when I felt my life had little purpose and I was just so unhappy. Do you have those days when you don't know where the time goes and by the end of the week you have no idea what you've done with your time? You have no idea why the week panned out like it did? That was me through and through.

Then, I had to deal with an awful breakup and ended up feeling completely worthless. I finally reached my breaking point. I was sitting on the train thinking to myself: *Is this it? Is this what life is? Going from one thing to the next, trying to make every day work and feeling lousy at the end of it.* I was stressed from balancing school with work, and I felt displaced at university and uncomfortable in the environment away from home. All of these together had me feeling really unsettled and anxious and I didn't have a clue what to do. Yes, I could call my parents any time I wanted, and my best friend was always there for me, but it's the internal feeling of anxiety that is hard to shift. It's got nothing to do with anyone else, it's a feeling inside you. It's hard to explain—you just don't feel right. For so long my confidence and self-esteem had been at an all-time low and all I could focus on were the negative elements of my life rather than the positives. It was hard and I often look back at that time and wonder how the hell I got through it. The answer is that all of this stress triggered the first "why" that drove me toward the gym.

It was on a journey home from work one day that my "why" came to me. I was on the train when I had a lightbulb moment: I decided enough was enough and I needed to get a grip and take control. Why? Because I am responsible for my happiness and my health and I wanted to feel strong, energized and able. So, what did I do? I took my first step into the gym, signed up for a twelve-month membership and, well, the rest is history...kind of!

Signing up for that gym membership was definitely the beginning of my fitness journey, but the truth is it took me two months to actually step foot inside that gym again. I'd taken the first step to sign up and get my life in order, but by the time I got back home, life got in the way—again. I got busy with work and school, everything felt like a blur again and the stress started to creep up. I know I'm not the only person to have felt this way. We all suffer from the same pressure and anxiety, and as much as we all experience it in different ways, there is a reason we all relate to one another:

we feel like other things and situations are controlling us and all we want is to be in control, to be confident in our decisions and to feel good about ourselves.

I realized that as much as I worried about everything, I had no control over the level of work I needed to do for school or the fact that I had to keep working to live. Somewhere along the way I recalled the gym membership I hadn't used for a few months. I realized the gym was something I could control. Working out and training was new, it was something I could escape to. It was slightly daunting and I felt nervous about walking into a new environment, but unlike the stress of work, relationships and school, I realized every single time I had managed to work out over the years, I actually felt good. Part of me was also excited. It felt good to put on workout clothes, and I sort of made an "event" of going to the gym. I planned it in advance and I knew it was happening, so part of me was actually looking forward to it—it was about to break up the monotony of my day and I was excited to try something new. The only way is up with fitness and exercise, and I needed that release, that strength and that confidence. For the sake of my mental and emotional health, I needed to train and I needed to make fitness a habit—that was my "why."

I remember walking into the gym, finding the weights section and trying to figure out how to use the leg press machine—it looked like something from the movie *Transformers*. Every time I had been to the gym before, or even done PE at school, I used to run and do a bit of cardio here and there, but it was the weights that really interested me. As I approached the leg press machine, I didn't focus on my anxiety, I focused on understanding and learning how to use this new piece of equipment. Don't get me wrong, I was scared. I was nervous people were staring, thinking I didn't have a clue what I was doing. But, once I asked for a bit of help and started to learn more, I noticed everyone is there for themselves; everyone focuses on their own goals and they all have their own "why." That first workout was the best feeling—the only feeling, in that moment—and it helped me forget about my worries and anxieties and made me stronger.

I learned, I asked questions, I researched and kept practicing. Something that seemed so complicated actually became simple in theory and truly energizing in practice. It was a game changer for me. I felt strong, confident and powerful. Most important, training allowed me to focus, and it allowed me to channel my energy and time into something that was good for me. And, like I said before, it gave me something to look forward to during the day. I didn't dread the long lectures or shifts at work because I also had something in my schedule that was helping me in myself. Always start with you as your "why." Training is your time. Every part of the exercise and experience is to do with your mind and your body—how you move, what you can do, what you want to do—and that's why it's such an empowering part of your "why." You're literally doing it for you.

Once I started training more regularly, another "why" emerged. I used training to help me stay sharp in lectures when I was at university. Not long after I started attending the gym, I realized I was more switched on in my lectures. It was a "why" I hadn't anticipated but the effect was profound and I stuck with it. If I didn't train, my mental capacity wasn't what it should have been. When I had a two-hour lecture, I struggled to be present and take on board the information I needed; I felt tired and sluggish and lacked concentration. Once exercise became a part of my daily routine, those lectures felt so much more manageable. The energy I expended in the gym flowed over into my university work and, in the same way I'd wanted to succeed and smash it in the gym, I wanted the same for my lectures. I wanted to take it all in, to use the information I was being taught to get smarter. I'd switch off my phone in order to focus and be totally present, as I knew the progress I was making in the gym could be applied at university too. In fact, there is now masses of research to suggest exercise is beneficial for learning—your memory improves, as does your ability to think and reason, and regular exercise helps to stimulate the growth of cells in the brain.[2] Tell your parents, kids or partner that and I'm sure you'll all start working out together!

I was also so much happier when I trained. I felt so good after each workout, I felt positive and motivated, and my family and friends could see and feel that too. Exercise releases endorphins, which help to reduce feelings of pain, anxiety and stress. It makes you happy and less likely to feel stressed and worried. So my "why" was for me but it had a positive impact on others in my life too. It made me stronger and better for others, and made me realize I wanted to help other people achieve their goals.

When I started my Instagram account, the happiness and satisfaction I felt when someone sent me a message to say they'd worked out, they'd joined the gym, they'd made time to train just because of what they saw on my platform was truly inspiring. They inspired me. The community of amazing women that I was building kept me going. We may be training in isolation, but we are also training as a community to be better, to do better for ourselves. That's my final "why": to help, support and show women how to be their own "why," their own reason and their own goals. That gets me up in the morning and that makes me sleep well at night.

My "whys" are ingrained in me and I look back at them a lot. From when I first started training up until today, I have discovered new "whys," my priorities have changed and my focus has shifted. The same might happen for you as you progress on your fitness journey. It's important to check in regularly and keep asking yourself, "why?" Revisit, rethink and revise.

No matter what, I make sure my "whys" are clear, to the point and simple—and that's exactly what yours should be too:

- I train because it makes me feel strong and confident.
- I train because it makes me happy.
- I train because it relaxes me—it's my therapy.
- I train because I like the routine and structure it adds to my life.
- I train because it keeps me accountable and focused.

HOW TO FIND YOUR "WHY"

YOUR "WHY" IS the foundation of your journey, the reason you jump out of bed, the reason you keep pushing yourself to do the extra set, complete the extra mile and keep coming back. Without your "why," your purpose and reason, healthy habits, routines, discipline and consistency will fizzle out before you've even completed your free trial at the gym!

Take a minute, sit back, and ask yourself—why have you picked up this book? Why are you reading it? I hope it has something to do with your desire to be a better version of yourself, to evaluate and change up your fitness and health routines, to make *you* a priority. So many women struggle

DO THIS FOR YOU

to put themselves first because they think it's selfish; they feel guilty for prioritizing themselves and making time for themselves above others, whether that be loved ones or work. I don't think putting yourself first is selfish; you need to allow it to feel necessary and positive. It's self-love, self-care, meaning you are ever evolving with the power and confidence to always do what works for you.

I know finding your "why" is not as simple as saying or starting with the words "health" and "happiness." For so many of us, our "why" is rooted in other people—children, parents, partners, loved ones. However, your happiness cannot be rooted in other people. Yes, you love them, they matter, they are important and necessary parts of your life. BUT, you cannot be the best person for them if you're not the best person for yourself. To be fully present, happy and healthy for them, you have to start with you, and this is exactly where your "why" for your fitness journey needs to start.

By applying this principle to your personal goals, you can discover what truly drives you, and that will be the foundation on which you build a healthy lifestyle.

WHY FITNESS?

PEOPLE DON'T BELIEVE me when I say fitness changed my life. They think I'm being over the top, exaggerating or that somehow it comes easily to me. It isn't easy and I'm not exaggerating. Fitness came to me at a challenging time and has had the greatest, most positive impact on me.

In the past, most of us have been taught to see working out as a physical benefit. Our doctors tell us it's good for us, and the positives highlighted are usually all related to physical health:

- Bone and joint health
- Heart health
- An increase in stamina
- Less risk of injury and disease
- Likely to live a longer life

You might expect me to focus solely on the physical benefits of exercise. However, I truly believe it is as much about the mental and emotional ones. My work ethic, schedule, discipline, resilience and consistency all come from fitness. I cannot emphasize that enough. I truly mean it when I say it has changed all areas of my life. It puts me in a good mood; it wakes me up; it gives structure to my day; it keeps me focused; it's my therapy, my stress relief and, above all, fitness makes me happy.

BE CAREFUL OF CERTAIN "WHYS"

WHEN I WAS getting into the swing of things with my training, like so many people, I wasn't just training to relieve my stress and help me feel better, I was focused on my aesthetic goal—in my case I really wanted "a bigger booty." I had seen pictures of what I thought was a desirable body and that's what I wanted. I was going to the gym because I loved it, but I also wanted that curvier physique. But, the more I chased it, the more stressed I got. The more I looked at myself in the mirror after every training session, the more disheartened I felt. It didn't stop me from going to the gym (I was slowly developing the discipline, patience and habits to exercise), but it did leave me feeling annoyed and frustrated. It was almost making me impatient.

The problem with an aesthetic "why" is it takes you out of your head. It makes you focus on short-term goals and you're more likely to give up or slow down and be inconsistent. You start to focus on what you can see as opposed to how you feel. When I started my journey and my community began to grow, people were sharing their progress pictures and they were sending me messages about their progress with their squats or weights, but that wasn't their "why" or the thing that really spurred them on to keep going. What kept them going was the inner strength, the mindset, the habits and the fact that they felt more confident, happy and more present with themselves, their friends and family. Don't get me wrong, I love training glutes, I love a strong back, I love an ab workout (sometimes!) and I love seeing the results. I know you will probably have an aesthetic "why"—we all do—and it's natural to care about our appearance. We all have hang-ups or things we'd like to change about our bodies. That's perfectly normal. BUT try not to make it your primary "why." Dig deeper and find something that drives you mentally and emotionally. Your primary "why" needs to be focused on how it makes you feel, how it benefits you—not just what you see in the mirror.

So many people are successful in their careers, but feel unfulfilled. So many people are lean or "ripped," but feel depressed. So many have loads of friends, but feel lonely. Your "why" isn't about what you see in the mirror—it needs to be about how it makes you be the very best version of yourself.

Fitness is also a source of independence. It gives you the

time and space to do things just for you. Fitness is an internal process as much as it is an external one. It teaches you so much more than you think it will. If you really embrace it and see it as an integral part of your lifestyle, you'll become your own priority, you'll grow stronger and better for yourself and, in turn, for everyone else around you. You'll learn patience, discipline, resilience, confidence—the benefits are almost endless.

If you can enter the alien environment of the gym or a new class or try a new sport and persevere, you're showing yourself you can succeed and that feeling is addictive. Once you've proved to yourself you can succeed once—whether that's through a class, a long run or hitting a personal best when you squat—you won't be as daunted by another experience, by trying something else new. You'll have learned in the gym what perseverance can do for you and you'll take that into every other walk of life.

When you're in a space where you feel self-confident, that's when you feel like you can deal with whatever comes your way and when you can implement healthy habits that will stay with you for a lifetime. By identifying your "why" and reminding yourself of it time and time again, you will learn to overcome the obstacles and excuses that prevent you from being your best self.

TASK: LIST YOUR "WHYS"

The first thing I want you to do is grab a pen and paper then write down why you are embracing fitness and a healthy lifestyle from this moment onward.

It could be a list of things like mine (see page 11) or just a few sentences. There is no right or wrong, except your "why" is totally to do with you. We all have our reasons, and they often start with an aesthetic goal. If that's true for you, then I want you try to think of the mental aspect of what you're reaching toward. Perhaps, for example, you want to lose weight to fit into your wedding dress. As much as that might be true, your real why is actually to feel confident, to smile, to be happy in your own skin on your wedding day.

I want you to write down your "why" but I want you to think about the difference it makes to your mind and body. Think about how you want to feel, what you want for yourself. Get it down on paper so you always have it to look back on. When you're feeling low or unmotivated, your "why" will come through, trust me—I live and breathe it!

Your list of reasons why is solely for you, but I want you to monitor the positive impact they have on those around you. I get it: loved ones, work, friends, everything around you is important. But, I want you to remember that, by prioritizing your health and fitness and your reasons for wanting to smash a workout, you will be a better person for everyone else too. People will feel your energy, they'll love your strength and they'll admire you for it too. Don't be afraid of putting yourself first, ever!

CHAPTER 2

LOSE THE EXCUSES

You've figured out your "why" or you're well on your way to understanding why you are getting fit and healthy, but, if it was that easy, everyone would be doing it and I wouldn't be writing this book! So, what gets in the way of that drive to smash a workout, to eat healthily, to reach your goals? Excuses.

We make excuses every day. Think about it: the sleeping in that means you skip a workout, the takeout that means you don't need to cook. We need to recognize excuses (no matter how big or small) for what they are, stop giving them the power that they have and learn how to deal with them.

I CAN'T...

EXCUSES TURN CHALLENGES, fears and nerves into a phrase I hate: "I can't."

- I can't work out tonight because everyone at work is going for drinks, and I can't say no.

- I can't clean the bathroom because I don't have the time because of work.
- I can't do a pull-up and I'll never be able to because I can't commit to going to the gym that much.

This language is negative. It's dull. It's unnecessary. Instead of starting with "I can't," which of course gives our excuses and limitations power over us, you need to think about what you can and will do.

- I can go for drinks as soon as I've completed this workout and I'll have so much more energy to talk to all my colleagues.
- I will wake up a little earlier to clean the bathroom and I will feel so much better once it's done.
- I can go to the gym and work out at home three times per week and I'll focus on exercises that will help me do a pull-up in good time.

This language is motivating; it's way more positive and, I don't know about you, but it puts me in a good mood. Exercise has shown me this is possible. I've walked up to the squat rack not having a clue how to hold a barbell and within a few weeks I was squatting set after set after set. That can-do attitude is addictive, believe me!

MAYBE LATER...

I'M FAR FROM perfect. I have those times when I'm sitting down and chilling but I haven't worked out—those are the moments when it's easy to start looking for an excuse:

- Should I make myself a coffee?
- I'll just spend five minutes browsing through my phone. (It's never five minutes, by the way....)
- I'll go in the morning as I'll have more energy then.

Procrastination is a beast. I struggled with it as a student and I'm sure you or your friends and family are guilty of falling into this trap. Everything seems way more appealing when you're procrastinating, but before you know it, hours have passed and the guilt and regret of not accomplishing much begins to sink in. You start to kick yourself and ask yourself why you didn't manage to get the workout in, or the essay done or the to-do list ticked off.

But if you start asking yourself why you decided to procrastinate, I'd say you're asking yourself the wrong question. Procrastination is a valid feeling, but it's usually because the task at hand isn't right. If you decided you were going to go on a 5k run after work, but have never really run more than 2k, plus you're absolutely shattered every day after a long commute, there is a glaring problem with your actual task. Similarly, if you want to run a half marathon and you know it's creeping up on you, you're less likely to prepare for it if you just keep thinking about the full distance you have to run. And let me tell you, that would put me off too!

So break it down. Change your schedule and put more manageable routines in place. Instead of that 5k, make time in your schedule to run 3k, three times a week before work, so that you're not exhausted by the commute before you have even started. Instead of thinking about the half marathon as one long distance, start with a shorter distance and make a plan to run a little further each time. Make your tasks fit your routine, so you will be less likely to procrastinate.

Having said that, all of us will end up procrastinating at one time or another. When you do, my top tip is to act like you're running on a 10 percent battery. When momentum starts to die down, treat your work like a "red light" battery warning. You have less than 10 percent to get all your stuff done before your phone dies. You will surprise yourself with how much you can fit in when you tune into "battery dying" mode. It works!

What else could you do in these moments? Jump up, grab your gym gear and get moving straight away. I learned not to give myself the headspace to think of excuses. There are times when I am thinking, "I can't be bothered," but I have trained my mind and body to work against the word "can't." I always do the opposite—I get up and get moving.

I KNOW, BUT...

THIS EXCUSE ALWAYS makes me laugh. You try to explain why your excuse is valid and reasonable, even though you've just admitted there is no reason for an excuse!

- I know I should go for a run, but it's raining.
- I know I should cook myself a healthy meal, but fast food is so much easier.
- I know I should clean the bathroom, but I can always do it tomorrow.

These are the types of excuses that will make you unhappy because you know they're excuses—you'll feel bad about not working out, or eating yet more fast food, and you'll feel frustrated when you come back to a bathroom that still needs to be cleaned. What's more, they'll play on your mind all day because you know they were excuses and you know you wanted the opposite.

In these instances, you need to try to switch up the way you think about the situation. Like I said earlier, just change the language and remember your "why." Your "why," whether it's a nice clean and fresh house (which is a workout in itself, by the way), or smashing a 30-minute workout, will get you through. You just need to shift your focus away from the "but" and back toward your "why."

I DON'T KNOW HOW

ANOTHER TYPE OF excuse is the one where you think it's beyond you; that you can't do the task at hand because you don't know how to do it and you'll somehow get it wrong, it won't go to plan or you'll look silly.

This "fear of failure" is the simplest but toughest mindset to beat because it's ingrained in all of us. I think it's bigger than just an excuse as it can affect the way you think about everything—home, work, life and relationships. And over time I've realized it has something to do with how we react to change. We avoid change and seem to fear what's new so we replace it with excuses:

- I don't know how or when I'd find time to work out because I'm so busy already.
- I don't know what to buy to eat healthily and I don't know what it will taste like.
- I don't know if my grades will be good enough.

But where does this blocker come from? It's like a brick wall: you say you can't do something or you don't know how to do it and resort to your comfort zone. Yet that comfort zone isn't making you happy in the first place. You feel tired, bored, unconfident and unmotivated, so why do we fear changing it so much?

The truth is, we're scared of the potential failure because putting ourselves out there is a risk and makes us vulnerable; we might reveal so-called weaknesses, gaps or things about us that make us feel unconfident. Instead, we choose to stick to the comfortable option because it is what we know. Comfort zones are, of course, comfortable—but so is your sofa and you can't spend your whole life there. It's important not to see our weaknesses as "weak"; they are opportunities for us to learn and do more. Challenges and the unknown are uncomfortable, but this is where we learn to grow.

I had no idea what to do at the gym or how to cook healthily in the kitchen when I first started. My mom's warm and hearty Albanian recipes were all I knew so for a couple of months I did just stick to those. After a while I realized that I was using a fear of failure and change as an excuse, so I made the time to learn about nutrition and balanced eating. Did I get everything right the first time? No. Was it scary, uncomfortable and at times really annoying? Yes. I got so much wrong. However, as I kept going I discovered that it was in fact the failures that I was learning from. It is only through trying, failing and trying again that we can grow.

Children and young people are so much more used to learning. When you're a child you are doing and experiencing things for the first time, whether that be reading your first book or having your first argument with your best friend. Emotionally, mentally and physically, you're learning every day. When you become an adult, it's not that you stop being able to learn new things, it's that you get comfortable with established routines and lifestyles. For a lot of us, it is during this time when new fears and comfort zones develop.

We create excuses to stay as we are as it can seem like so much effort to make a change. You're tired after work, you're exhausted by the time the weekend rolls in, you're "fine" with the way things are. But, in reality, you're not. You're just used to the feelings of frustration and unhappiness and you've started to believe that this is how things should be. And that's where the excuses come from. I'm here to tell you: you're wrong and that's not how things need to be. Your life, your body and your health can be in the exact shape you want them to be because *you* control them. They don't control you!

Think about the last time you learned a new skill, such as baking a cake, learning a new language or even hanging wallpaper. Did it feel good? We need to rediscover a love of learning to take away the fear of failure. We need to embrace new challenges, be excited and not shy away from them; that's when these excuses will end and real change will begin.

NOT TODAY

SOME EXCUSES ARE legitimate, but it's vital we reevaluate them often. Examples include:

- I can't work out because I'm injured.
- I can't make it to the gym because I have a deadline to meet at work.
- I can't meet my friend because I need to save some money.

These can't be constant excuses; they're a one-off. They come through feelings of urgency, importance and circumstances. The best way to overcome these hurdles is through listing and organizing your weeks, days and months ahead to help you prepare and preempt these curveballs (I will look at this in more detail in Chapter 3, see page 35). That way, you'll still be in control of your time and, therefore, have power over your excuses.

Excuses, in whatever guise they come, can be self-debilitating and can stop you reaching your goals. If you believe them, they can give you the impression they're real. They're not. So whenever you are faced with an excuse, remember this: training can always be adapted to suit you and your circumstances. You just have to make the time.

TASK: FLIP YOUR EXCUSES

Excuses will derail you and take over if you let them; good intentions are meaningless if you give in to your excuses. Instead, do what I do and flip your excuses into action:

- *I can't go for a run because it's raining* becomes: I'm going to do a 20-minute high-intensity workout indoors because it's raining.

- *I said I would meet my colleague for a drink after work so I won't have time to work out* becomes: I'll get my workout in at lunchtime or before work so I can meet up with my colleague after work.

I want you to list five excuses you commonly make to avoid working out. Now, like I've done above, flip them around and turn them into a positive action instead.

HURDLES AND BARRIERS

THERE ARE CERTAIN things that aren't excuses, just facts of life. They are more like barriers or hurdles, which get in the way of our routines, schedules and habits, and there isn't much we can do about them. I am not a doctor, but I couldn't write a book without including what I want women to be aware of when it comes to their health and fitness journeys. Women are strong and powerful. We endure a lot, from growing up in a male-dominated world, to experiencing things like:

- Menstruation
- Hormone imbalances
- Menopause
- Endometriosis
- Pregnancy

…and so much more that only a medical expert can advise you on. Our bodies and minds go through a lot. Needless to say, these things are not excuses, they are facts of life and ones that can make us feel isolated and unsupported. I am here for you. I may not have all the answers, but I will support you and make sure we overcome these challenges together so you can live your life feeling healthy and fit.

Your period

It might be wrong to call a woman's menstrual cycle a hurdle but, let's be honest, it can be really annoying! For so many of us, periods can be uncomfortable, painful and make us just want to stay in bed. I totally get it. For years as a teenager,

I had the most uncomfortable periods; I would want to stay home from school because the pain would make me feel sick, my skin was awful and I'd want to cry all the time. Then, when I was put on the pill to try to manage my periods, I just felt sick all the time, I was so bloated and I started to suffer with acne. It was horrible. The bloating was the worst…I know I'm not the only one who suffers with it.

In my opinion, the relationship between menstruation and exercise needs to be spoken about more. Of course we can keep training—and exercise can be really good for you at your time of the month—but that doesn't help women (especially teenagers) with common issues such as:

- Stomach cramps
- Headaches
- Tender breasts
- Bloating
- Mood swings
- Tiredness
- Diet (I want *all* the chocolate)
- Skin issues

When you first start your periods, it can take time to settle into a regular cycle. Although this is completely normal, it can really mess with your daily routine. Then, when they do start to settle, you might decide to take the contraceptive pill, which can disrupt your cycle even more. If you start college or a new job, the stress of that life change can affect your cycle, too. Plus, when your period is due and you are feeling bloated, lethargic and not your best, sometimes the last thing you want to do is put on gym leggings or shorts to work out.

I totally get it, I've been through all of this and I've come out the other end. First thing to remember is your progesterone and estrogen levels are low during your period, which leads to feeling tired and low on energy. This is completely normal and why you might feel less inclined to work out. The lack of these hormones also might leave you feeling achy, more prone to headaches and emotional too. As much as all of this is real and truly affects so many of us, I want to get rid of the stigma surrounding our periods. Yes, it's something we can't avoid, but that doesn't mean we need to stop getting on with our lives for a couple of weeks a month. You need the energy and you need to beat the pain—exercise can help! It can give you more energy and lift your mood by releasing endorphins, the body's "feel-good" chemicals, which can really help beat the blues. Exercise can also help beat the pain caused by cramps and backache, too.

There may also be other hormonal imbalances that can affect your training regime, diet and emotional well-being, but exercise—whether it be a daily walk or a 45-minute strength session—can really help you manage and overcome these hurdles. You can totally do this and let your workouts help you along the way!

You can try to overcome the hurdles through:

Opting for lower-intensity exercises. Try steady state cardio (see page 140) for the lower body and focus more on resistance work for your upper body.

Drinking water and staying hydrated. Water can really help beat the bloat, flush out your system and keep you energized during your period.

Eating lots of fruit, vegetables and fiber. The tiredness and low hormone levels can make you crave sugary food—as much as you want it, it will just make you feel tired and increase the bloat.

Keeping track of your cycle. By planning your workouts mindfully according to your cycle, you can adjust the intensity or length of your workouts during your period. As it's planned, you know it still fits with your routine, reducing the stress around it.

Sleeping. Rest well during the night so you have the energy for your workouts.

Although a hurdle, your period doesn't have to stop you in your tracks. With prior planning it can be managed so that you learn to work around it and keep on training. Soon enough, your attitude toward your period and your capability during that time will change, and you will no longer see it as a hurdle.

Menopause

Another "hurdle" that isn't spoken about nearly enough is menopause as well as premature menopause. Menopause usually affects women over the age of 45, but premature menopause can occur in women younger than that. Menopause is when a woman stops having periods. Women may experience mood swings, sleeplessness, hot flashes, weight gain, and many other symptoms. There is a lot more research needed into this stage in a woman's life and it's definitely something we should all be aware of. You might not be nearing menopause, but perhaps your mom or someone else you love is going through it and could do with your support. At this stage, as much as women might want to work out, they might not feel like they can or have the energy to. Here are some tips for ways in which you can still sustain a fit and healthy life with exercise at this stage too:

A daily walk. Walking outside and getting some fresh air gives you energy and keeps you in a focused routine. It is your time to focus on yourself or maybe listen to a podcast while staying fit too. If you don't feel like going outside, you can try the treadmill in the gym or even the crosstrainer or stairmaster for some steady state cardio to keep you fit, healthy and active.

Light resistance work. Osteoporosis and aches and pains in your body are more likely and common in menopause. Using light weights or resistance bands can help strengthen your bones, joints and muscles to alleviate these pains.

Swimming. It's refreshing, it's good for your mind and body, and it's relaxing.

Try maintaining a level of fitness on a daily basis as it will really help with your mood and energy, which will help you manage the symptoms of menopause.

Endometriosis

Endometriosis is a chronic inflammatory condition where tissue grows outside the uterus, mainly within the pelvic areas (ovaries, fallopian tubes and around the uterus). It can leave women struggling on a month-to-month basis with cramps, sickness, tiredness and sometimes fertility problems. It can be a real struggle for so many women and I really feel for you if you have been diagnosed with it. However, you are strong and capable and, when you feel you can, exercise and following a balanced diet can improve your well-being. Seek medical help and do as much research as you can to help you with the condition—you don't need to let it stop you feeling in control. Endometriosis is a challenge and one that can be worrying, but with the right help and support, you can tackle it.

Pregnancy

Pregnancy is seen as a major hurdle in a woman's fitness journey. So many women will stop training or be scared of training simply because they don't know what to do or where to get advice. Well, I am here to help as much as I can.

If you are pregnant, you first need to get clearance from your doctor that you are fit to train. That is extremely important as only your doctor will be able to check and confirm that you are okay to exercise. Once you've been given the okay, it's time to address some of the common questions we get:

IS IT SAFE FOR ME TO WORK OUT IF I'M PREGNANT?

If your doctor has given you the all-clear, it's safe for you to train. Pregnancy is a sensitive time in a woman's life for so many reasons—most of all, you're growing a human! Your body will go through so many changes, mentally, emotionally and physically. Your hormone balance changes, your mood changes, your energy levels change—everything changes! Change can make you and your loved ones run back to safety, put your feet up, rest for nine months and just take care of the baby. If your doctor has given you the all-clear, they will also advise you on the type of exercise you can do during your pregnancy. Like I always say, we're all different, pregnant or not, so do follow the particular advice you have been given by your doctor and midwife. Exercise *is* taking care of you and your baby, but it goes without saying: see how you do. Every stage of your pregnancy is different; listen to your body and do workouts that feel right. It might be a brisk walk or even a resistance session—just listen to your body.

CAN I TRAIN WITH WEIGHTS IF I'M PREGNANT?

Now this is a tricky one and, again, it depends on the medical advice you've been given and your training experience. If you've used weights before, you should be fine to keep training with weights during your pregnancy too. However, you need to be careful with the amount of weight you are lifting and how you are performing different exercises. My best advice would be to train with a qualified prenatal trainer or to follow a prenatal workout guide. There isn't any research or evidence to rule out weight training completely when pregnant, but you just need to be mindful of a couple of things:

- The hormone relaxin relaxes your ligaments, especially in your pelvis and lower body, to prepare you to push the baby out. Because of this, you may find that you can stretch a little further or you might feel a little more flexible than usual. You need to be mindful of all exercise, not just strength and resistance training, as you may find you strain your back or pull a muscle more easily without noticing, all because of the relaxin running through your body.

- The baby needs to grow in your belly, which means your abdominal muscles will need to relax—do not worry, this is completely natural! Many women worry about losing their abs or gaining a "mum tum" but changes to your tummy are completely natural when you're growing a human. That's amazing! You'll need to avoid traditional ab exercises like full planks, crunches, full push-ups, mountain climbers and so on. Substitute these for exercises that help strengthen your deep core and pelvic muscles. Pilates is a really good workout, or consult a prenatal personal trainer to guide you through the right exercises. Most exercises can be modified with appropriate core engagement, like push-ups and planks on your knees, for example.

HOW MUCH SHOULD I EXERCISE IN EACH TRIMESTER?

This will vary from woman to woman. Go with how you feel. They say you may feel quite tired in the first trimester, energetic in the second, and ready to pop in your third! Some exercise on a daily basis, even a brisk walk, is beneficial for you and baby, as long as your doctor and trainer say so. Go with what feels right for you, your baby, and your health.

WHAT KIND OF EXERCISE CAN I DO IN PREGNANCY? IS THERE ANYTHING I SHOULD AVOID?

Apart from contact and extreme sports (football, basketball, rock climbing, kayaking…), most exercise, under the guidance of a specialist, should be fine. Swimming and walking are great. As mentioned earlier, be mindful of how much you are lifting if you are strength training, especially as the pregnancy develops—remember, the baby is a weight in itself! Modify your ab workouts too. There is some research to suggest that lying down on your back for too long isn't recommended.[1] Like I always say, exercise is for life and it needs to work with your lifestyle. So, during your pregnancy, work on strengthening your upper body so you can feed and carry the baby with ease; strengthen your quads and glutes as you'll be changing diapers down on the floor and crawling around after your little one within months! Go with what feels right for your body and always, always consult a prenatal specialist for more guidance.

Pelvic floor work (Kegel exercises) is always good, so make sure you engage and exercise your pelvic floor muscles throughout and after your pregnancy. (In fact, it's important for all women in all stages of life to do these exercises.) When referring to our pelvic floor muscles, we usually point toward our lower abdominal muscles. While these are important, our specific pelvic floor muscles sit at the base of these core abdominal muscles; they control our ability to pass urine and feces and they sit around our vagina, urethra and anus. Here's how to exercise them:

1. Sit or stand comfortably (a Pilates ball is great for this).
2. Take a nice big deep breath in, letting your pelvic floor muscles relax.
3. As you breathe out, engage your abdominal muscles as if they are coming up behind your belly button.
4. Contract your Kegel muscles (the muscles surrounding your vagina) as if you are pulling them

up—it will feel like you are drawing them to a close. Bear in mind: don't clench your glutes, this is the wrong feeling for this exercise.

5. Hold for 5–10 seconds, release and repeat 10–15 times. Do this every day, or as many times as you like.

WHEN CAN I START TRAINING AGAIN AFTER LABOR?

The doctor's advice is usually six weeks. But, please don't rush back. You've just had a baby, a beautiful bundle of joy. You've been through labor, which is a challenge in itself. Rest, recover and you'll get back into the swing of things in no time.

Remember that every pregnancy is different and it is also an ever-changing state. You might feel perfectly fine throughout your pregnancy, you might have times when you have no energy to exercise, or you may have medical reasons why you can't train. Whatever the hurdle or barrier, you can manage it and overcome it. Fitness will always be here for you, so long as you know to seek the advice and guidance you need from professionals to help you overcome these challenges.

CHAPTER 3

MAXIMIZE YOUR TIME

When Michelle Obama was First Lady of the United States of America, she'd set her alarm for 4:30 am so she could squeeze in a workout before her daughters, Malia and Sasha, woke up. The woman with arguably one of the most hectic and demanding schedules in the modern world could find time for exercise. Why? Because she prioritized herself, which in turn made her a better mother, wife and First Lady. And if Michelle can find time, you can find time.

Whenever I train anyone, one of the most common excuses I come across is that people don't have *time* to work out. The reality is that's not the case and, if they want to, everyone can find the time. It comes down to what your priorities are. If you are not making time to eat well and work out, then you don't feel your best, you're simply not putting yourself first and not managing your time well—it's as simple as that. Remember, you come first and only then will you have the time to care for others with full energy and concentration.

We all have the time, we just choose how we spend it, and, for some of us, self-care, fitness and health just isn't part of that choice. Make it a priority, change the way you think, organize your time and it will change your life forever. We all wear many different hats in our lives—students, parents, workers, partners, friends, caregivers, daughters, sisters— all of us have to be a lot of things for a lot of people. I was working thirty hours a week while a full-time university student and I still managed to find the time to work out around three times a week—sometimes more, sometimes less. I promise you, I'm far from superhuman, it just all came down to how I organized my time, ignored the excuses and made myself a priority.

MAKING TIME

I BET A PORTION of your current week is spent doing unnecessary things or reserved for other people—if you can find time for them, you can find time for yourself. I'll also guarantee a portion of your time is spent doing things you could switch up to find time to exercise. Don't get me wrong, I get it that we all have other very important things or people in our lives and, more often than not, those seem like the *only* important thing. If you have children, they come first; if you have a demanding job, there are deadlines to meet; if you're taking care of your parents, their needs come first; if you have a pet (like my gorgeous dog, Buttons), they need time too. I totally get it. But, you must remember that there is *always* time for you—you just have to adjust your mindset, believe that you're worth it and make it happen.

Put your phone away

Go grab your phone. Go into your settings and take a look at your average weekly screen time report. Apparently, the average adult spends 34 years looking at a screen over their lifetime…*34 years!*[1] Given the way our lives work now, I'm assuming much of that has to do with work, which can't really be helped. We use computers, phones, laptops, tablets, TV— no wonder so many of us feel addicted. But I also bet a big portion of that time is spent scrolling on social media, watching videos, online shopping—basically, anything that lets us zone out for a while. My work is heavily rooted in online media, and I love it, but so is my lifestyle. I use social media to see what my friends are getting up to and to keep in touch with my Tone & Sculpt community and family. Social media is also how I keep up to date with recent news, current trends and, of course, all the Tone & Sculpt updates. Every day I ask myself: has the time spent online today been completely productive or beneficial for me? I'll be honest, the answer is usually, no. I will usually waste some portion of my day mindlessly scrolling on my phone. What would your answer be?

Mindless scrolling and streaming services are everyone's first choice because they're comfortable and easy. After a long day at work, or if you've got five minutes to yourself, nothing seems more comforting than passively scrolling. We sit, we chill and we scroll. We watch. We relax. But, let's be honest, it's just not healthy. I know we say it's a bit of zoning-out time, and I totally get that, but if you want to focus on you and do this for you, that will not come from so much leisure time in front of screens. Put your phone down, tune into your body and try these tips to stop you from endlessly scrolling and checking your phone:

- Charge your phone away from the bedroom so that it is not the first thing you check in the morning.
- Buy a separate alarm clock so you don't need to rely on your phone.
- Try to avoid using your phone for an hour after you wake up or before you go to sleep—plan a tech-free morning and bedtime routine.
- Try setting aside only fifteen to twenty minutes a day to mindlessly scroll. This way you won't feel like doing it all day long.
- Replace scrolling and checking your phone with reading a book or newspaper.
- Listen to podcasts when going for a walk.

Instead of scrolling through your phone, switch on your favorite playlist and do some squats, jumping jacks, stretching—move your body and notice how much more energized, positive and motivated you feel. And trust me, you'll sleep better too! Yes, there is a time and place for sitting back, relaxing and losing yourself in a box set or book (I prefer a book). But, if that's what you're doing most of the time, this is where you make time to move your body, plan meals and feel great about the healthy lifestyle you're forming.

We all have commitments and I know a lot of us are guilty of only ever putting other people first, but in order to truly understand what self-care is, you must make the time for it. Self-care isn't just about downloading the app, buying the book or signing up to the class. It's committing. It's respecting your mind and body enough to say to yourself, "I care about you, and I'm going to make time for you because you deserve it." The power in respecting yourself is huge and the confidence that comes with it is just transformational.

If your schedule is as packed as Michelle Obama's, take a page out of her book and set your alarm that little bit earlier to squeeze in some "me time" before your day starts. *The early bird catches the worm,* is that how the phrase goes? In a nutshell, make time by waking up that little bit earlier and going to bed a little earlier too. Replace your late-night film with meal prep, movement or some extra shut-eye. It doesn't have to be an hour and it doesn't have to involve a drive to the gym—you can do twenty minutes in your family room or yard, or get some steps in while you walk the dog. Just make time for yourself a priority. When you prioritize yourself and start to care for *you*, beautiful, seismic changes can happen.

TASK: PLAN YOUR WEEK

I use the calendar on my phone to schedule my entire life. Every Sunday night or Monday morning, I sit down with my to-do list for the week and plan my time: meetings, dog walks, meal prep, workouts…I don't go as far as bathroom breaks but it is nearly that much detail. I plan my meals and my exercises so that I remove the question of what I'm doing when. It means that even during my busiest weeks, I am able to maintain a healthy lifestyle. Now it's your turn to do the same.

1. Take out your calendar, to-do list or whatever you use to organize your time and make a list of everything you have to do this week that will get in the way of training and cooking healthily.
2. Find time around these things to schedule in a quick workout and some meal prep and write it into your calendar. You are more likely to do it if it is scheduled.

3. Better yet, is there anything you could change on your to-do list and schedule that will make training and self-care a bit more doable for you?
4. Go through your calendar again and swap out irrelevant unnecessary tasks (even if it's only five minutes) for movement and exercise. And write it down! If it's in your schedule, you are more likely to do it.

WHY MAKE TIME TO WORK OUT?

YOU'D HAVE TO have been living on the moon to ignore the fitness revolution of the last twenty years. J. Lo's doing it, Michelle's doing it, I'm doing it! You know deep down that to get up and move your body is unbelievably good for you. The sooner you start to have a healthy relationship with your own body and exercise routine, all areas of your life will improve, so now is the time to make time.

This is when excuses (see Chapter 2) start to feed in again: I don't have time, I can't find the time—this will only be true if you let it. Remember, you have to *make* the time. I'm not saying this book alone will rid your mind of excuses. What I am saying is train your mind to channel that energy into doing something positive for you. Always remember that an excuse provides a short-term win, like having an extra ten minutes of mindless scrolling or leaving the bathroom to be cleaned until next week. However, an action provides a long-term win, long-term progress—that ten-minute workout will lead to more energy, better habits and a willingness to do more for yourself. The positive energy will radiate from you and you will be a better person for you and those around you.

It takes time

I am asked time and time again, "How do you find the time? You must be superwoman!" I'm not. No one is and don't let anyone tell you they are—like you and me, they are normal people, they just take control of their time and they are stronger and healthier for it. They are also patient. If you have the patience and discipline to enjoy and persevere with this journey, you will go far. Everything takes time, and with time you need patience too—something that needs constant practice and constant reassurance.

When I learned to be patient with myself, to be patient with my journey, to learn the discipline to keep going, I realized things were becoming more consistent; things were falling into place. I was on my way to forming healthy habits—the most important part of any fitness and health journey.

CHAPTER 4

FORM HEALTHY HABITS

Telomeres are like the ends of cotton buds; they are little caps at the ends of our chromosomes that protect them when our cells divide. Telomeres get a little shorter each time a cell divides. Essentially, telomeres determine how quickly we age and how quickly our cells decay and die. Put quite simply, we want to preserve our telomeres to live a long and fruitful life! So, how do we do that? Research suggests that telomeres age with stress, anxiety and a sedentary lifestyle. There is now more and more research that strongly points to exercise and a healthy lifestyle slowing the aging and decaying process of telomeres.[1] In other words, making fitness and your health a habit early on in life will lead to a long and prosperous one! Fitness is not a quick fix and it is not a novelty. I have not and will never advocate a 21-day transformation because you cannot place a time limit on a healthy habit, which is essentially what fitness should be.

Fitness should be ingrained in your schedule. For me, it is in my calendar like any other appointment or reminder, and we know you wouldn't think to cancel or simply not turn up for the dentist or hairdresser because you don't want to let them down. Make an appointment with yourself, with your exercise mat, the gym, wherever it is you choose to work out, and make it a habit—don't let yourself down either.

The definition of a habit is "a settled or regular tendency or practice, especially one that is hard to give up." I'd add a little change to this definition: habits are ingrained into our routines and lifestyles; they are challenging to forge and equally difficult to give up. Turning fitness and exercise into a habit will soon mean you can't give them up!

If you start seeing fitness as a switch you flip, it will soon become an ingrained habit. It will become a habit that you put into your schedule without even thinking twice about it, a habit that will make you feel better and better each and every day. You don't think about brushing your teeth twice a day and that's how we need to get you looking at fitness. At first, parents have to train and remind their children to brush their teeth, explaining the benefits and the consequences of not doing it. They have dentists and advertising to help them. You have *me*, this book, your friends, family and an awesome community out there supporting and reminding you that fitness is a healthy habit—one that you cannot and should not be without.

HOW LONG DOES IT TAKE FOR FITNESS TO BECOME A HABIT?

SCIENCE WILL TELL you it takes twenty-one days to form a habit, but that's not entirely accurate. The truth about habit formation is that it'll take *at least* three weeks, likely longer, depending on the habit you're trying to form.

The twenty-one-day idea came from a cosmetic surgeon in the 1950s; he noticed it was taking his patients around twenty-one days to get used to seeing their new faces or their new nose as their reflection. Similarly, with amputations, he noticed it took roughly the same amount of time for patients to accept their limb was gone—they'd sense the phantom limb for around three weeks before accepting their new situation. In 1960, the surgeon in question, Maxwell Maltz, wrote a book about his findings, entitled *Psycho-Cybernetics.*[2] It sold 30 million copies and scientists generally accepted it takes three weeks to form a new habit. But a UK study from University College London in 2009 found that on average it takes more than two months to form a habit, with some subjects in the study taking 254 days for the habit to form.[3] My point is that you can't put a time limit on habitual learning and that way of thinking may deter you from your goal and journey.

What if I told you it took three weeks and you got to day 22 and didn't feel it was a habit? Would you give up? Would you stop following me and jump on the next trend that promised you a quick result? I hope not. I hope what you would realize is that habitual behavior and learning takes time and differs from person to person. The key lesson is to be consistent and keep going.

The universally accepted truth is that if you do something enough times, it will become a habit—simple math! It won't happen overnight, but it's worth considering that in the University College London study, some participants found habits formed after just eighteen days. Every journey is individual so there's no right or wrong in terms of how long it takes you to form a habit. You are on your own journey and that is all that matters. What's important is that you consciously stick to the routine for as long as you need to for it to become a habit.

If you want fitness to be a habit, you need to do it frequently until it feels like second nature. There might be days when you don't feel like it but on those days you have to remind yourself that this is a journey and you're working to form a habit to be the best version of yourself. I have "bad" days, but when I do, I get up and move. It's a habit: my innate reaction to lethargy is to completely reverse the feeling and move. It's an instinct in me and something I now don't even have to think about—but remember, it hasn't magically become a habit, I've *made* it a habit.

People look at me and think I *love* working out and, therefore, it comes easily to me. They assume that motivation is somehow a natural inclination of mine. It's not. I was just like you, knowing I should work out but not really knowing what to do or having the motivation to do it. I hope you have nothing but good days, but I'm sure there will also be bad days when your motivation is low. It is on the bad days when forming a habit becomes super-important; we cannot rely on motivation but we can rely on our habits—they are ingrained!

Drinking water is something we know should be a habit, but for many of us it's not something we really like to do. I don't know about you, but I'd much rather be drinking a chocolate milkshake every hour than desperately trying to get to the bottom of a two-liter bottle of pure H_2O! But, I also know that, compared to that chocolate milkshake, water is good for my energy levels, my muscles, my bones, my skin and so much more. I remind myself of the benefits, the reasons (my "whys") and it keeps me going. Lesson number one to form healthy habits? Remind yourself why you are building them and why they are good for you.

What's important in habit formation is how you view the habit. You're trying to create healthy changes that you'll sustain for the rest of your life. You might have picked up this book because you want a smaller waist or to shift a few pounds and, while I understand that is something you want, I also want you to remember healthy habits lead to a healthy, fulfilling lifestyle. A strong and powerful body will last you way longer and make you happier in the long run than inches off your waist in time for a vacation.

HOW TO FORM HEALTHY HABITS

CHARLES DUHIGG IS one of my favorite authors. In his book *The Power of Habit*,[4] he sets out a structure that the majority of our habits follow, whether we're brushing our teeth or eating chocolate: cue, routine and reward. For example, our stomach rumbling (cue) may cause us to reach for a snack (routine) and then we feel satiated (reward). The research around habits suggests that the more we notice the cues, follow the routines and benefit from the rewards, the less brain power is used to think about these habits and the more likely we are to do them—they become ingrained. Now imagine using the same theory for your workout.

When at university, I was falling into a spiral of bad habits: if I was hungry, I would reach for chocolate or junk food; whenever my alarm went off, my inconsistent sleeping patterns would cause me to hit the snooze button so many times that I'd end up rushing out of the door, completely disorganized and stressed. These were habits, but unhealthy ones that needed to change. The danger of habits, good or bad, is that they are just as challenging to unlearn as they are to learn.

Let's think back to my "why," my excuses and my use of time. I was getting to a stage where stress and anxiety were really starting to take over. Any little thing—running out of coffee, forgetting to text my friends back, being late for work—would set me off and I'd either cry or want to run away. I was at breaking point and needed a change in my life. Habit formation is successful if you believe in yourself and you feel that you can truly make that change to become your best self. And I did. I knew the process and journey were not going to be easy, but I wanted to be happier, healthier and confident, all of which can be learned by forming healthy habits. This is what I did:

- On Sundays, I would meal prep for the week and put food in individual containers in the fridge.
- I would pack my gym bag the night before a workout or wear my gym gear in the morning (school was casual, so I could get away with it).
- I would schedule my workouts for the week at the same time every day and set an alarm on my phone to remind me of them.
- I would write a routine before heading to the gym.
- I would always carry a bottle of water.
- My bag was packed with loads of healthy snacks to keep me going during lectures.
- I reduced my scrolling and social media time.
- Where possible, I would walk instead of drive or take public transport.

As well as all of this, I forced myself not to give in to excuses by changing my language. Remember, we don't say *I can't*, we always say *I can* and *I will*. And I did.

Before I knew it, meal prep, getting to and from the gym, drinking water, everything became second nature. Not only this, but I was seeing and *feeling* the difference. I was more energized, more alert, more organized and I had more time. It is such a gift to have free time after a busy day of lectures, work, the gym and socializing—and I only uncovered this free time once I had made a habit of exercise. Plus, my legs were shaping up and I was pretty happy about that too! For some it takes 21 days and for others 254, but overall, habit formation will happen with the right mindset, willpower and drive to do better for *you*.

TASK: GET ORGANIZED

Write down the small things you can do on a daily basis to make sure you get that workout in. It could be:

- Make sure your lunch is ready the night before.
- Pack your gym bag the night before.
- Set out your workout gear and mat ready for the morning.
- Buy a two-liter water bottle.
- Schedule the time of day you will work out every day.

Remember, not every workout needs to be a two-hour gym session—mine definitely aren't. Work with your lifestyle, your personality and your "why." What makes you happy? Why do you want to work out? Maybe it's training to run a

5k, in which case do a 10–20 minute run a few times a week. Maybe you want to improve your posture, so do a mobility workout every day and back training at the gym. If you carry a bottle of water around with you all day, you'll find you drink more water than if you had to get up and get a glass of water every time you're thirsty. In order for healthy habits to form, you need to make it as easy as possible. You need to remove the barriers, the obstacles and the excuses that have prevented you changing before.

Whatever it is, do what works for you, as there is no competition, no rush—just consistency, willpower and perseverance.

Fitness for me is as much a necessity as eating or sleeping and that's where we need you to get to. You need to feel it's as much a nourishment for your body as eating is; that it's vital for your existence, because it is. When I walked into that gym for the very first time, I had no idea it would change my entire life and career. But I know it soon felt like I didn't want a life that didn't have fitness in it. It gave me so much more than I had to give it in return. In exchange for a bit of sweat and hard work, I felt brighter, better, more focused, fitter, healthier, more rested; I felt all those benefits from just a few consistent sessions a week.

You need to look at what fitness is *giving* you, not what it's *taking* from you. In exchange for a bit of time, you'll get back so much more than you ever put in.

HOW TO SHIFT BAD HABITS

INTERESTINGLY, BUT PERHAPS unsurprisingly, the word "habit" can also have negative connotations. Smoking, drinking, biting your nails—they are all bad habits. But for some reason, we keep going with them—they are things we enjoy even though we know they are bad for us. Now I'm all about balance, but smoking is a bad habit and it is not good for your health. It's addictive and it's an addiction you need to kick if you're a smoker. How do you kick the habit? Discipline, taking steps to stop, being consistent and forcing yourself to make a change. Sometimes, especially when you continue to do something that isn't good for you, you just have to force yourself to stop. You keep telling yourself to stop, you tell others to tell you to stop and you need to keep reminding yourself of your "why." Habits are something we do all the time; we learn to enjoy them or find them comfortable and therapeutic. They just "feel good" even if, in reality, they're bad for us, so we are the only ones who can make the change to shift a bad habit.

On the other hand, working out is good for you, but is seen as a chore, something we have to work really hard at to fit into our day. Why don't we see it as something to look forward to, something that we do consistently, on a daily basis, around the same time (if that works for you), something that is a part of a successful daily routine? Well, you *can* see it that way and you *will*—as I've said before, all you need to do is change your mindset. And, trust me, you'll feel a damn sight better after your workout than you will after a cigarette!

Hand on heart, I see exercise as just as much an enjoyable part of my day or week as getting a massage or a facial. It might not always have been like that, but it is now. Just writing about working out makes me want to get my gym gear on and crack out half an hour of training—but I won't because working out has also taught me discipline!

You need to change the language you use to work out. Instead of saying, "I *need* to work out," say, "I *want* to." Instead of saying, "I still have a workout to do," say, "I can't wait to get to the gym!" Working out is awesome: it's beauty, it's strength, it's you time, it's self-care. I remind myself that working out is my time to shine. It's my time to show what I can do. It's time for me to build on yesterday, last week. It's picking up where I left off and getting better and better every single time. It's taking the baton and running with it. It's improving. It's showing up and moving forward every single session.

However, working out and forming a healthy habit is still a choice as much as shifting a bad habit: smoking, going for that tub of ice cream and biting your nails. It is a choice that only you can make and a habit only you can change. When trying to shift a bad habit, try to remember the following:

- You are replacing it with a healthy routine, one that will make you feel better and that is in line with your goals and your "why."
- You have the willpower to do so; you just need to keep reminding yourself.
- You have the right support network and community to keep you accountable and make sure you stick to it.

I am here to help you, the Tone & Sculpt community is here to support you, your friends, family, loved ones, and colleagues are here for you. Everyone you trust will have your best interests at heart, and that's what will shift the bad habits so you stick to the healthy ones.

HOW DO I STICK TO HEALTHY HABITS?

EVERYONE HAS THOSE days where they're not feeling it, and as much as habits are hard to break once formed, sometimes good, habitual behavior can come to an end. If you sincerely follow the steps and thought processes outlined so far this will be unlikely, but life happens and I am mindful of that.

Forming habits should take out feelings of apathy but that doesn't mean I'm not susceptible to wanting to sleep in and skip the gym occasionally; we're all human, after all, and sustaining habits can be just as challenging as making them.

There might be those friends who judge you or make you feel awkward for choosing your workout over a drink with them. Maybe you have a partner who just isn't ready yet to make the same commitment and finds it weird that you choose to go to the gym when you could have a nice evening in. The guilt or pressure, whatever you want to call it, can be challenging to deal with and sometimes it's just easier to say, "I'll just get the workout in when I'm free." Perhaps you work in a very high-pressure environment with long hours and leaving work a little earlier three times a week just isn't an option—we all know the world of work is trying to catch up with the importance of health and fitness in our lives. Or, maybe you work from home. So many workplaces are now all for flexible working, and the conversation about working from home is becoming so much more acceptable—and so it should! When I started my company, I wanted my team to feel like work fit into their lifestyle—I didn't want them to fit into mine. We can only work and be at full capacity if we take time out for ourselves and a workout is just that. So if you do have the option of working from home, use the time when you would otherwise be commuting to fit in a 20-minute bodyweight session, or go to the gym. The temptation to sleep in is real, but your day will feel so much more amazing if you fit in a workout—it's about taking control of your time and doing something for you!

I'm here to encourage you to make exercise a part of your life, but I know the major impact lifestyle can have on making fitness a habit. It's not necessarily your choice, but your situation can take its toll on putting yourself first. When this happens and you feel the urge to just "skip" today, think back to Chapters 1 and 2: always remember your "why" and always work through the steps on how to overcome your barriers and excuses. You have to keep going and remember why you started in the first place and what you want to achieve. Like with work, school and life in general, fitness is a skill; habit formation is a skill. It takes patience, commitment and learning, so from time to time, you will have to revisit those first steps and remind yourself how to start and why you need to keep going.

When apathy strikes, you need to focus on your "why" and the cues that will get you up and moving:

- Put your favorite track on and start with a dance to warm you up.
- If dancing isn't your thing, try skipping. We all know how to do it and it'll get you moving in the same way dancing will—as a gentle warm-up.
- Stretch out the stress, tension and anxiety to get you ready and roaring for your workout.
- Put your gym gear on. Trust me, it is the cue you need to kick-start your workout.

- Watch or look up a new routine to smash at home or at the gym.

Just start. Just. Keep. Showing. Up. That's all any of us can do. Keep showing up again and again and again. Keep trying and the rest will follow, I promise.

In those moments of apathy, don't put an expectation on how long you'll be exercising for or how many pounds you're going to squat. Just start. Start and see where it takes you. Workouts often have a momentum and a mind of their own, similar to those nights out when you think you can't be bothered to go. It's when we expect the least that we sometimes end up surprising ourselves the most. Keep reminding yourself that you'll never regret it. How can you regret doing something so good for you? You know you won't, so just start.

All these examples and thoughts are about shifting your mindset so you see working out exactly like any other lifestyle habit. It's about finding time for you in your busy life and viewing that time as non-negotiable. My workouts are such a lifeline for me: not only do they keep me fit, healthy and feeling strong, they're also the time in my day when I can step away from all the other things I have to do—the emails I have to return, the calls I have to make, the work I have to finish. They're literally the best part of my day.

NEAT

HAVE YOU HEARD of NEAT? It stands for non-exercise activity thermogenesis, which basically means the movement you do on a daily basis, like taking the stairs, cleaning or running around after your kids. You might even do NEAT at work, especially if you have a job that involves a lot of movement. NEAT can even be part of your commute if you walk for some of it. You don't need to train vigorously every day, but I do think you should get some movement every day. Plus, NEAT is a great way to start making fitness a habit and to start seeing fitness as a part of your lifestyle too.

We've probably all heard of the global target of 10,000 steps a day. In fact, this is what makes so many of us count our steps and buy fitness trackers. I'm not saying fitness trackers are a bad thing at all, I just don't want a number to dictate how you feel about fitness. The million dollar question is: *do you have to walk 10,000 steps a day?* The first time I got asked this I had to do a bit of research because I've always just gone with the 10,000 figure without really thinking about it. The question made me revisit everything I cover about healthy habits throughout the book—why am I putting a number on my achievement on a daily basis? Where has this figure come from? Apparently, the number was once part of a marketing campaign for the Tokyo Olympics in 1964.[5] It was for the sale of a pedometer called Manpo-kei, which means "10,000 steps meter." Apparently, since then, it's kind of stuck with all of us. The research suggests that yes, if you're managing 10,000 steps a day you are active—I mean, that's pretty obvious. But then, just like I said with forming healthy habits, there is research to suggest 5,500 steps is better than 10,000 steps, 4,000 steps is a good target to reach too…even better, 15,000 steps. Do you notice a pattern? The number shouldn't matter—stop focusing on a number and focus on what *you* can achieve and do. What fits in with *your lifestyle* until it becomes a healthy habit for you.

For example, if you're a student, you're going to be sitting in lectures a lot and studying a lot so why not take the stairs to lectures, walk to class, and take a break from your desk every now and again to do a few stretches or a few squats? The same applies if you have a desk job. If you have kids, you're bound to be running around after them a lot, changing diapers, and crawling up and down slides with them! That is all activity and a big feature of NEAT—nothing really to do with steps. But, make sure you're stretching and releasing some of the stress that might come with running around after the kids all day. There are so many ways of making movement a habit and because this is something that is literally a part of your lifestyle, you'll find movement and fitness increasing in no time. Why not try:

- Taking the stairs
- Walking instead of driving
- Cleaning
- Gardening
- Playing around with your kids and friends—and rediscovering that childhood love for activity.

If you're in retail, teaching, or have an active job, you're bound to be keeping your NEAT and stamina up every day. Movement is good for you and it should feature in your lifestyle on a daily basis. Once you get used to this, incorporating the gym or a more vigorous workout will become second nature—vigorous exercise is still recommended to work all your muscles, get your blood flowing and increase your strength and stamina. NEAT and exercise work hand in hand and, by treating movement holistically as a habit, you're more likely to fit it into your routine and make it a habit for life.

HEALTHY HABITS FOR LIFE

WOMEN GO THROUGH so many changes in their lives, physically and hormonally, from puberty to pregnancy to menopause. Our physical state fluctuates and can change our bone density, energy levels and hormone levels. Working out will help you regulate so much more than your aesthetic appearance. Forming healthy habits for life gives you discipline and makes you more resilient to change. Why? Because exercise becomes the constant "comfort zone" in your life that you can control. It's your time and you can adapt your workouts to work with your lifestyle choices and changes. If we want to keep working out for life, let's take a look at a few of the benefits we'll feel every decade we decide to keep working out.

Teens

Most teens are still doing some form of exercise at school. With hormones all over the place during the difficult teenage years, exercise and working out has been found to be a mood stabilizer. Exercise increases self-esteem, reduces the risk of depression, promotes sleep and builds self-confidence—all the things teenagers so desperately need. If we start exercising when we are younger, we are more likely to maintain a healthy and balanced approach to food and fitness as we get older[6]. We learn so many of our habits as we grow up, so learning to adopt a lifestyle that includes exercise when we are young will only make adulthood better. Going to the gym or working out at home will be second nature.

Twenties

A large study conducted between 1985 and 2011 found that those who started exercising in their twenties reduced their risk of illness and disease in later life.[7] Your twenties are most likely the decade when you're not the kindest to your body too—late nights out, a bad diet, burning the candle at both ends. That's fine for a while—you're young and your body will take it. But it's worth remembering that your twenties, as well as being the most hedonistic time of your life, are also the prime time to strengthen bone and build muscle. You're not growing anymore but your bones can still grow in density. Strength training will help with bone density in your twenties and will stand you in fantastic stead when you're older.

Thirties

Hormonal changes in your thirties make it slightly tougher to build bone density but resistance training will make sure you don't lose any of the bone density you already have. Working out in your thirties will lower your risk of type-2 diabetes, high blood pressure and high cholesterol.

Forties

Working out in your forties can add years to your life. Exercise will support posture if you're working at a desk, hunching over children or just slouching without knowing. Perimenopause can start in your forties and keeping bones dense and strong will help to protect against osteoporosis.

Fifties

Once you reach your sixth decade, you start losing muscle mass. However, regular exercise helps maintain it. You may need longer to recover in between workouts, but in addition to helping your body stay strong, exercise in your fifties will also help maintain brain health.

Sixties and over

In addition to preventing diseases ranging from heart disease to diabetes, studies have found working out regularly in your senior years improves your immune system. Regular exercise—including strength and resistance work—from your sixties onward also improves strength and flexibility, which is vital due to the increased risk of falls once you reach older age.

Decades and age aside, exercise is a form of stress relief, mindfulness and purpose. It gives your emotional and physical health something to focus on. Exercise as a habit in itself is something you need to sustain to stay positive, stay healthy and be the best version of yourself. The habit itself will become its own motivation. Just remember your cues, stick to your routine and keep at it. The rewards will radiate from you!

CHAPTER 5

SHIFT YOUR
PERSPECTIVE

As a society we have become target driven. From school to work, it's about looking forward, aiming for something, getting somewhere. We are given targets and goals at school, then in our careers and in our personal lives too! What grades did you get? What fitness plan are you following? Where are you applying for jobs? When's your next promotion due? And the one that gets to me the most: are you in a relationship yet? Do you have children? We like a metric; we like to see how many hours a month we're working out. We like to know we're "on track."

Targets are not necessarily a bad thing. They keep us focused, they keep us going and they give us something to look forward to. However, the problem is we've become obsessed with reaching the next stage, setting yet another goal, so much so that there has been a stark rise in anxiety and stress levels. In fact, if we are feeling stressed or anxious, we are often told to set a goal to beat procrastination, to shift the mindset. I'm not going to quote numbers or research here, just turn the news on, or check online—the stress and anxiety associated with achievement is everywhere. My problem with specific goals and targets—whether it's aiming for a personal best in your squat, doing a hundred burpees (why even would you?!), or losing twenty pounds—is that you can lose perspective and, actually, you gain nothing.

GOALS

I KNOW WE PERHAPS need goals in different areas of life, but I really don't like the word "goals" when it comes to fitness. It's a term that's bandied about so much and, frankly, I find it cheesy and misleading. Even SMART goals. SMART stands for Specific, Measurable, Achievable, Relevant and Time-bound goals. The idea is that you set yourself an achievable goal, keeping in mind your current context and reality so that you can ensure the target is specific, measurable and can be achieved within a period of time. For example:

> I will run a 5k race in six weeks. I will train for it by running three times a week on a Tuesday, Thursday and Saturday for the next six weeks. I will start off by running for twenty minutes and I will add on five minutes' worth of running time every week. I will use my smart watch to measure my distance and my aim is to run the full 5k by week five.

But the goal is still focused on the end achievement. What happens after the race? Do you stop running consistently three times a week? Do you then panic and worry about your next goal? Or do you celebrate your achievement (which, of course, you should) and think you're done with fitness for a while? I think goals and targets are what put so many women off making fitness a lifelong habit because they always think it is something to "fulfill and complete."

Fitness should be a lifelong, sustainable habit to stay healthy, moving and happy. It should not be based on a picture that you want to "be" or a number on the scale; they mean nothing unless you are enjoying the journey and appreciating all of the other benefits that come from exercise. Think back to what I said about counting steps in Chapter 4—a focus on a number can of course be "motivating" but it's short lived and can be disheartening if you don't reach that target. You're less likely to turn it into a habit if you just focus on a number.

Say my imaginary friend Sarah gave herself a goal of losing twenty pounds before she goes on vacation in three months—you might say with the "right" calorie deficit, exercise schedule and willpower, it's an achievable goal and her reward is the vacation in three months. But it's unsustainable if Sarah thinks she just needs to stop eating her favorite foods, stop eating out to avoid temptation and that she *must* work out for a set time each week, even if life happens. What happens if she has a deadline at work to meet, a friend from out of town turns up whom she hasn't seen in months, or she falls ill? Does this mean she's failed? Does this make fitness unachievable? Well, if Sarah has a goal of losing twenty pounds with a rigid plan that clearly doesn't work with her lifestyle, then yes, she will feel like she's failed. And what happens? Like many women, she stops, thinks fitness isn't for her and, like we covered in Chapter 2 (see page 17), she thinks she simply "can't" do it.

That goal doesn't take into account any of the reasons Sarah wants, or even needs, to lose twenty pounds. It's tunnel vision, singular in purpose. It doesn't have space to take into account why Sarah has this particular goal in mind or whether she's happy. It doesn't factor in the fact Sarah might be a mom of two with a full-time job who struggles to make ends meet and find time to work out. It doesn't take into account that maybe Sarah is a bit unhappy with where her life is at right now; it doesn't take into account that maybe, just maybe, this twenty-pound goal is based on something Sarah has seen or read, thinking if it works for someone else, it must be right for her. Setting a twenty-pound goal for Sarah is pointless because it's just about a single point in the future; it's an aesthetic goal that ignores so much more of her life and ignores the journey too. Sarah cannot confidently move forward with that singular point of weight loss as a focus until she looks at many other aspects of her life and accepts how she got there, why she supposedly needs to lose twenty pounds, and whether it's actually going to make her happy.

Let's go one step further. It might be that Sarah does manage to lose the twenty pounds, feels great, and enjoys her vacation. Then what? Like many who go on vacation, she returns having gained ten pounds and with no vacation to look forward to, she goes back to old habits, which eventually means she puts on the weight she had lost. What's the problem here? Sarah is just focusing on what she achieved and, now, what she has let go. At no point in this story is there a focus on the journey.

Goal setting can be a gimmick, as it puts forward a vision that ignores the process needed to get there and everything that you learn, become and achieve along the way. It doesn't take into account that the "small wins"—the organic changes along the way—are what we need to celebrate, love and appreciate. If you only focus on the destination, you'll miss so much of the journey and that's where the learning happens and where the healthy habits are formed.

Of course, I'm not saying goals aren't *real* and a time limit is a bad thing; all I'm saying is we need to change the way we look at them. We all have big goals, from training for different health reasons, to finishing a course or running a marathon. They do keep us on track and they are things that we should accomplish and feel proud of. But, I don't just want you to focus on the final goal. My point is, focus on everything along the way and be proud of the entire journey. Time limits can be helpful, especially if you're the type of person who likes working to a certain deadline or there is a challenge you've entered, like a 10k race, and you need to make sure you'll be able to run 10k by the date of the race. This is when a time limit is relevant, but don't put a limit on your journey. It is ongoing and forever evolving.

My "why," to get strong, fit, healthy, happy, to help others achieve the same in their lives, does not include numbers, it doesn't have targets. What it has are feelings, I feel strong, I feel fit. I have a healthy approach to food. I am happy. And I am determined to help others achieve the same in a lifestyle that suits them.

REFRAME YOUR THINKING

TOO OFTEN IN life, we focus on the destination rather than the journey. We make the target a six pack or a dress size rather than incrementally increasing how many sets or reps we can do or how much we can lift. We often ignore the fact we've overcome so much and learned so much on the journey to fitness—leaving behind relationships or jobs that weren't right for us and growing in confidence and mental strength as we continue to grow in physical strength. I want you to shift the focus from your goal or target and start celebrating everything you do along the way that makes you the very best version of yourself.

The journey is much better than the destination when it comes to so many things in life—and fitness is no different. If you focus on an end target, you'll have missed so much of the vital process along the way: the times when you didn't think you could finish the class but you did and you loved it; the times when you weren't sure you could get that final squat done but you smashed it and felt stronger than you ever thought possible; the times when you did your longest skipping session or run; the times when you'll look back at what you've achieved so far and realize the "old" you who started would never have thought this possible.

None of those things are the destination when you start off but they become important as you pass them by. If you only focus on an end goal, you'll miss so much of the process you go through to get there—how hard you work, the boundaries you've put in place, the habits you're working so hard to establish. . . . *All* of that is the journey and none of it is the destination. It's so important to observe and respect those processes.

Think about when a child throws their trash in the garbage can or says please or thank you for the first time. Think about the new song you discover and love on your drive to work. Think about the person who asked if you're okay today or the trainer who said you're doing wonderfully. That is what we need to celebrate. That is what we need to smile about, be happy about. That is life! I'm not saying you need to have a house party or spend tons of money to reward yourself each time (but it would be pretty cool if we could do that too!). What I am saying is you need to reframe your thinking to celebrate you and love you. That's what fitness is all about. If you are healthy, happy and feeling better and better every day—that is success.

TASK: SCRUTINIZE YOUR GOALS

Write down any goals you have set for yourself in relation to your fitness and health. Whatever your goals, think about the following:

- Is this goal a habit I want to sustain?
- How is it going to add value to my life?
- Is it going to make me happy?
- Does it have longevity?
- What do I think is going to happen when I reach my goal?

If the answer to any of these questions makes you feel uncertain, or the goal all of a sudden becomes unmotivating (I can't imagine any of us will be happy tracking our weight every day for the prospect of a life without chocolate!), you need to rethink, reframe and focus on the journey instead.

MINDFULNESS

REFRAMING IS A technique that is used a lot in mental health therapies and is often part of cognitive behavioral therapy (CBT). It's something we can all do in order to see other perspectives and possible feelings about things we thought were set in stone. You could say another term for it is being mindful. You are no doubt familiar with mindfulness; it has been a well-being buzzword for years and focuses on being present, being really in the moment of whatever you're doing and however you're doing it. For me, mindfulness is about acknowledging, accepting and being able to manage everything that's going on. That's my interpretation of it—I'm sure there are variations, but that's the beauty of making it work for you.

Mindful fitness is a newer phenomenon, which plays into what we're thinking about here. Mindful fitness is about being in the moment in the workout. It's not about a physical goal, it's about moving for health and well-being, about focusing on where you've come from, where you are presently and the journey you are on. It might be HIIT (high-intensity interval training), it might be spin or yoga or strength training—mindful fitness is about the process in your head when you're working out, not the workout itself. A mindful workout will have you focused, in the moment, really feeling each movement, your body and mind in clarity. It's about embracing the journey you're on rather than fixating on an endpoint.

For me, working out makes things less foggy. It gives me clarity and happiness; it's where my drive comes from. My best ideas for Tone & Sculpt and Oner Active have come in the vicinity of the squat rack, the treadmill, and my jump rope. When I talk about reframing, I'm talking about changing the way you look at things and reframing how you see them so your opinions become more balanced and you can train yourself to see things more positively and not just from a single point of view. Exercise has given me perspective and made me mindful of others and life in general.

Reframing is a difficult thing to do and it takes practice and continual effort but it's worth it, just like any workout. Once you know how to reframe your thoughts and feelings, change, habits and routine seem to settle in further too. Nothing is fixed and you realize so much more can be achieved.

Whenever we're presented with something, we all have an instant opinion—whether that's good, bad or somewhere in between. Thinking back to Chapter 2, it's where our excuses and barriers originate. Reframing not only gets you to think about things from a different perspective, but with time you'll start to become more in tune with your own opinions and you'll habitually question where they've come from, whether they're correct and how they've formed—whether it's a spur-of-the-moment opinion or something grounded in your background and upbringing.

A simple example of reframing comes back to how we view exercise. If we think back to Chapter 4 on habits, exercise is usually seen as a chore or an "extra" part of your day. But, if we commit to forming healthy habits and changing the way we view goals, we are ultimately reframing our thinking. That's the process I went through. I reframed what I'd always thought was the epitome of looking good and feeling great and now I feel at my best, my most incredible self, when I'm smashing it in the gym, not focusing on a particular image.

EMPATHY

LET'S ADD SOME perspective (after all, that is the title of the chapter). Be kind to yourself. Ultimately we're trying to change your relationship with exercise and that is a process and journey in itself. So far, I've effectively asked you to address a lot, from your mindset to habits to how you schedule your life. I empathize, so let's take a minute to celebrate how far you have come:

- You've thought about the healthy habits you want to form.
- You've reflected on your use of time and how to make it more productive and efficient.
- You're putting yourself first from now on.
- You're taking the time to read this book to be the best version of yourself.
- You've made a start.

That is all something to be celebrated and rewarded. You're fabulous!

While I want you ultimately to reframe the way you see your relationship with fitness, I find we see the best and worst in others before we see it in ourselves. We are quick to judge, to assume, to make excuses and put up barriers based on others and our environment. Let's reframe that.

Relative to what I said earlier, if you can see things from different perspectives, it's likely you have the ability to empathize with others in your life. If you can listen to someone else's perspective and feel grounded enough to appreciate their views even though they are not necessarily your own, it leads to such a healthy outlook on life. Some people practice grounding themselves in yoga. They breathe, they meditate. For me, these feelings of grounding, patience and resilience come from exercise. I have the patience to listen to my body and the discipline to keep going and I am constantly learning to focus on my progress in mind and body.

This is what exercise, routine and habitual behavior has taught me: if someone jumps the line in front of you, rather than a knee-jerk reaction and having a go at them, reframing might help you to see the action as an honest mistake they would happily rectify if you pointed it out to them. Reframing can give people the benefit of the doubt and in today's society, that's no bad thing, right? Equally, if they turn out to be someone in a rush or someone who just isn't bothered, don't let it bother you in the same way—overcome it. Like you would in a workout, no matter how much those muscles are burning, you take a deep breath, remember you're in control and stay focused.

Now if you can reframe your thinking, habit formation, cues, goal setting and celebration, reframing will become a positive force in your life. You'll feel buzzed about your workouts and you'll see them as something you value and love as much as getting your hair or nails done. You'll never miss the appointment with yourself and even when "life happens," you'll simply reschedule it and still get it done! Reframing will take time but it's something everyone can learn. If you've adopted some of the principles in this book already, you're well on your way to learning how to reframe successfully—most likely without even realizing it.

Put it in perspective: the workout isn't a means to an end. The workout is the end and it is the means. Healthy living has no end, it is ongoing. Always remember the journey is an ongoing process, one that does not end, but continues to grow, develop, prosper and complete you:

- You thought the workout was just to give you a beach body for a summer vacation?
  Reframe it: it's to make you fit and strong for life!

- You called chocolate a cheat food?
  Reframe it: in moderation, it is a healthy and positive part of your balanced lifestyle.

- You thought exercise means a gym membership?
  Reframe it: there are so many different ways to work out and feel strong that don't involve the gym.

TASK: REFRAME IT

I want you to reframe any limiting thoughts you have about exercise and healthy eating. Next time you're about to go to the gym or work out at home, rather than think of how tired you are or every other priority on your to-do list, reframe it: working out *is* a priority. *You are a priority.* You're looking forward to getting hot and sweaty, to getting stronger and fitter, to listening to your favorite playlist and doing your best.

Remember: motivation and excitement will fade, but habitual behavior and reframing your thinking won't.

A CHILD'S PERSPECTIVE

I ALWAYS LIKE TO look back, especially to childhood. People are all about moving forward, but, actually, looking back helps you move forward. It helps you evaluate lifelong habits and choices you've made and it gives you perspective; you can appreciate how far you have come while constantly making the necessary changes to keep you at your best.

Think about when you were a kid. How many times did your mom or dad tell you to slow down and not run? Did you ever walk down the stairs or did you jump down them a couple at a time, taking the last four in a huge leap? Did you stand still at break time or did you energetically run around the playground, playing games with your friends?

When you're a kid, movement is fun. We don't even *think* about standing still because there's too much chasing and racing around to be done. We cherish being out of breath and running around parks with our friends because it's so much fun. It's exciting; it's not a chore. Inherently as kids we loved moving and running and jumping and climbing.

Children see exercise—all exercise—as a laugh, as fun and something they can't wait to do. That is exactly how I want you to see exercise: a fun and beneficial part of life.

Ask a child why they're running around with their friends and they'll tell you it's because it's fun. Not because they need to do it. Kids are active. Their bodies want to move and run and climb—it's what we were built to do. But somehow we stop doing that when we get older and we see it as a chore to get back to—something we know we should do but can't always find or make the time for. So while I'm teaching you to reframe what you think about fitness, in essence what I'm partly asking you to do is rediscover that love of movement, the one all little kids have that disappears when we reach puberty or get a job and start "adulting."

There's so much we can learn from our younger selves when it comes to adopting a healthy relationship with the gym and fitness. Think about the trees you climbed as a child, the rope swings and the monkey bars. Did fear, failure or reluctance come to mind? No, because there wasn't anything to fear or fail at. Whatever you were doing wasn't about an end goal, it was just about the act of doing It. We wanted to see how far up the tree we could get so we'd keep climbing; we didn't fear how we'd get back down or what our parents would say (well, maybe a little). We just had fun.

Up to a certain age, children don't see failure in the same way adults do; for them it's all about learning. And if something doesn't seem to work out, well they just try again next time. They keep going, keep doing their best and learn along the way. It's only when they get older that they start to fear failure and maybe that's our fault as adults—life, responsibilities and this false necessity to achieve more and more kicks in.

Children's parameters aren't set in stone; they're more malleable than ours are. Children are used to trying new skills and adopting new things. They relish new opportunities. And what's more, when a child is self-conscious or worried about what others think, we as adults tell them to go for it! Not to care! Tapping into some of the emotions we had as children or even the advice we would give children can really help us push through some of the set thought patterns we've got as adults. Reframing the way you approach things and getting back some of that child-like wonder will help you massively on this journey—not only will you see challenges differently but you'll also start to see them as fun.

We become risk averse in adulthood, we stick to what we know rather than pushing ourselves in a different direction and we become staid and stuck, fearing change, resenting risk and preferring to stick with the status quo. But if you listen to those lessons from childhood, if you look back to that time, to who you were rather than just looking forward, you'll realize that risk isn't anything to be scared of, that sometimes the best things can happen when you take risks. Pushing yourself in a fitness and gym environment—using the machines you don't know about, asking for help when you don't know what you're doing, going into those traditionally male-dominated areas of the gym, stretching yourself in that controlled environment—will remind you of what you knew as a kid: that risk is good and can help you grow. It's one of the most important ways you will grow.

Once you realize that within a workout environment, you'll take it into your work and wider life. You won't fear change, you'll accept new challenges, you'll relish new opportunities and you'll grow because of it. And, like in childhood, the gym will become your release, your time to have fun, and putting on your gym gear will act as that break-time bell at school.

TASK: WRITE A LETTER

People always seem to suggest you write to your younger self. I want you to write to your adult self. Tell your adult self what you want to keep doing as you grow up, how you want to keep moving and how you're going to make sure you'll always be happy and healthy.

If you can see exercise as fun, if you can reframe your thinking and shift your perspective to see fitness and well-being in a positive way, all the benefits that come with regular exercise will be yours. Forming habits will be easier and the discipline and routine of exercising will become a fluid part of your lifestyle.

CHAPTER 6

BELIEVE YOU CAN

I spend a lot of time thinking about my journey and how far I've come and what I'm capable of now, which seemed like a pipe dream a few years ago. I look back at how scared and timid I was in the strength section of the gym when I first started going and wanted a "bigger booty." I reflect on everything I've accomplished along the way and that inspires me to kick on and keep going whenever I need it. If you could see me a few years ago in the gym, you wouldn't recognize me. I don't recognize me. I was scared of so many things, especially the male-dominated area of the gym. But I am so proud of that Krissy. I am proud of her as she took the steps to learn and build the confidence she needed to make me who I am today. It's taken time to get to where I am from where I started but I've focused on my journey and that's something I continue to do. I've learned to keep looking back every now and then to realize just how far I've come—that is where confidence is born.

My mom is one of the biggest inspirations of my life and whenever someone asks me about motivation and being confident in themselves, I think about her journey too. She moved here from Albania when I was a child and raised a family of four in a country and a language she didn't know. I had opportunities she could never have dreamed of; she worked day and night to make sure I did. She held our family together in tough times (and believe me, she's been through some tough times); she put food on our table, made with love, every single day. Her family has always been her priority, she's fiercely loyal and she doesn't care what other people think. She's gentle, tender, strong, fierce and caring. She's focused. As a mother, she wants what's best for me and she also wants me to be the best version of myself.

My mom has been one of the biggest supporters of my life, but she isn't one to sugarcoat things. She's honest with me and that honesty might not always be what I want to hear, but it's always what I need to hear. She's helped me get back up in times of need and she's my greatest supporter, but she makes me work hard too. Her life has been so incredibly different from mine, but when it comes to making sure I am a strong woman through and through, there are some valuable life lessons we can all learn from her:

- Trust your gut.
- Focus on your own journey and just keep going.
- Work hard and keep working hard. And just don't forget to work hard.
- Things take time and effort—nothing comes easy to anyone.
- People pleasing is normal, but please yourself first— know your own priorities and what matters most.
- Be yourself, your own superhero, your own inspiration.

- Be kind and humble. Always.
- Help others. Always.

When I designed my first fitness e-guide, I didn't expect anyone to buy it. I had no confidence that anyone would be interested—so many other ones were out there! But then they started selling. I called my mum and said, "Mum, I think one day I'll be able to buy you your own house." She responded, "Krissy, keep your feet close to the ground and stay humble, stay who you are because money will come and go but you and your heart have to remain how they have always been. A house can wait, you just keep doing you." She didn't care about the end goal. She doesn't rely on motivation or the opinions of others. She is her own source of confidence and grounding. And you can be too.

I've worked hard to be strong and self-confident. I used to apologize so much for my emotions and it really held me back. I was told so many times I was too aggressive in business so I'd apologize for being too direct, or saying too much or being too honest. But it felt wrong. I felt like people were trying to push back and make me something they wanted me to be as opposed to who I am. I stopped apologizing when I realized what people perceived as aggression was actually my passion, and I certainly wasn't going to apologize for feeling passionate about something I created and something I loved. The fact that my self-confidence came from within gave me the power to stop those apologies.

I'm also a big crier; I get emotional at all sorts of things, from films to family to when friends surprise me. I'd always apologize when the tears started to flow but I've stopped that now. Why should I minimize how I feel? The tears were a way of me expressing myself, not a sign of weakness or insecurity.

My self-esteem lets me revel in the tears that flow so easily, and I'm proud of how much I feel and how emotional I can be. In a world where so many people are repressed, I'm not. I have the liberty and the luxury to be confident, be the best version of myself and do what I love. That's freeing and it's powerful. Apologizing for who I am makes no sense, and it suggests I'm not complete or not good enough the way I am and it's self-limiting. Don't apologize for parts of your character that make you who you are.

CONFIDENCE FOR LIFE

LEARNING TO BE confident about who you are is tough and it won't happen overnight. But turning up for that workout, appreciating that you can dedicate five minutes, ten minutes, thirty minutes to work on yourself is a part of that journey to being and feeling confident in yourself. This is a journey and it's for life. Anything that promises overnight or short-term results isn't sustainable in the long term and will work against your confidence. Anything worth doing takes time and effort and we now know fitness shouldn't be a quick fix or an overnight success. I don't have any "quick fix" programs on the Tone & Sculpt app. The shortest program is four months, the longest can run into years. Why? Because anything that happens in a matter of weeks probably won't last months and the key to confidence is consistency, discipline and, yet again, healthy habits.

I've got so many friends who would hit the gym hard or crash diet before a vacation. Like "Sarah" (see page 63), they boarded that plane the size they wanted to be but after two weeks of cocktails and eating mindlessly, that hard work was undone. They may have had a goal and achieved the end target, but they were not consistent and, therefore, healthy habits and a consistent approach to fitness was yet to be achieved. You need consistency in order for any journey to be successful.

Think about buying a car. If you had all the money in the world but couldn't drive, what would you do first? Buy a really expensive car or learn to drive? My answer would be to learn to drive. But the temptation and excitement around a fancy new car trumps that practical thing and you buy the car on an impulse. What happens? You admire it while it sits on your driveway or in the garage taking up space. It won't bring you the happiness you thought it would because you don't know how to drive it. Like the dress that is a size smaller or the fancy gym membership you decide to invest in, none of it is worthwhile until you are consistent and disciplined with the time and habits needed to be able to benefit from it.

So where does the confidence fit in? Well, once you've passed your driving test, you become a better and better driver; the more miles you log, the more time you spend on the road, the more confidence you have. From the second you pass your test, you get better at driving. You also become more interested in cars and you learn more about them to make informed decisions on the type of car you want to drive. Plus, you end up enjoying the car more too. The same can be said for fitness: the more you train, the more consistent you are, the more interested and confident you'll become. The more you learn about fitness, the more streamlined and successful your workouts will be. And you'll enjoy it too! Working out becomes synonymous with jumping in the car to get from A to B.

When it comes to fitness, no matter who you are, your achievement should be rooted in your confidence, happiness and long-term health. Those three things are the only way to build a long-term relationship with fitness and exercise. You have to view your relationship with fitness and goals almost like an actual romantic relationship. It needs to be a relationship based on honoring your plans (your routine and habits), recognizing things aren't always easy (patience and discipline), knowing you're in this for the long haul (changing your lifestyle) and making sure it makes you happy (finding what works for you, day after day, month after month, year after year).

HOW DO I BECOME CONFIDENT?

GYM CONFIDENCE IS something you can be one hundred percent in charge of. If you go for a promotion and you don't get it, it's not necessarily because you did anything wrong, you just weren't the person for the job. When a relationship ends, it's not because there is anything wrong with you, the relationship just wasn't working. But the way that rejection can knock your confidence shouldn't be underestimated because the lack of control you had in that decision has an impact. When you work out, however, there's no one else to stop you achieving insane levels of confidence or success. *You* can persevere, *you* can affect the outcome, *you* can get the result you want, all with some hard work and determination. And, the more you work on yourself, the more you'll take any relationship- or work-related knocks on the chin!

The relationship you need to build with yourself in order to succeed and achieve and be your own inspiration is such an important one, and if you foster it properly, it'll be a relationship that's positive for the rest of your life. In order to do that though, you need to make sure you treat it like you would any other relationship and give it the care and attention it needs—all of which can be achieved in the time you dedicate to your personal workout. It's your breathing space, your headspace, your time to focus on you and show yourself what you're capable of!

So far, everything we have discussed means you're well on your way to being confident in your fitness routine. We have covered:

- Your "why" (Chapter 1)
- Beating excuses and barriers (Chapter 2)
- Managing your time (Chapter 3)
- Building healthy habits (Chapter 4)
- Reframing your thinking and having perspective (Chapter 5)

And now we know consistency, patience and discipline are integral to building confidence in fitness. Most of these things have been mental and emotional skills for us to develop. The next thing: community.

CHAPTER 7

FIND YOUR TRIBE

I am fortunate enough to have my social media familia and, like a real family, we support each other, help each other out, and don't always agree with one another, but we all care and we're all there for each other.

I know women sign up to the Tone & Sculpt app with a physical target but they stay for different reasons. I've had women buddy up and find friends and support each other from all over the world time-starved single moms and executives who motivate each other as part of a huge community of women who are changing their lives for the better.

While I don't want you to compare yourself to anyone— not the people in the gym, not the people you see online, not the transformation pictures you see—I do want you to find the people who bring out the best in you: the friends you have currently, the ones you're yet to make, the ones at your gym or spin class. They don't have to be gym buddies or people you work out with. I have a best friend who has always been there for me. She knows when to make me laugh, when to let me sob and when to kick my ass into gear. She helps me keep going when I need it. She helps me stand back up again when I fall down.

Like I said before, my mom is one of the most supportive people I know, but she doesn't get the concept of the gym. That's fine, I don't need her to, but her unwavering support is invaluable to me. Plus she's all about tough love and when it comes to fitness, tough love is what we all want from our trainers—and that's what I'm about to give you. Be part of a community, a group, a movement who push each other on, encourage one another to stay disciplined and, above all else, keep you accountable.

There are studies that prove a workout buddy is great for motivation in the gym. One study indicates that when we exercise with a partner, we tend to mimic their behaviour.[1] That's powerful. What that means is that if our partner is working hard and doing everything they can to get that workout done to the best of their ability, so will you! But your supporters don't need to physically stand next to you and do the same thing while you get your sweat on. We've all got friends who are into different things but we ask them about their love life or their hobby even though it's not something we do. Your friends that don't work out or do a different exercise from you can still be your supporters.

There's a massive "pack power," a powerful energy that comes from women supporting one another. I see it in the Tone & Sculpt community all the time. There are millions of us, all in a pack, all cresting a different point of a different wave in terms of where we are on our journey, and yet we're still looking out for each other constantly, ready to catch, cheer and spur the next person on. When someone in the familia says they're struggling, they're overwhelmed with support from women who've been in the same hole, the same rut; women who've felt the same way but have managed to move past it and keep going.

As individuals in the Tone & Sculpt familia, we have strength because we're all building confidence in our own journeys, but as a pack we have impact, we make a difference to other people—and that's huge. I've also learned from my Tone & Sculpt familia that seeing other women train is really motivating. They love that sense of community and being part of something, as opposed to feeling like they're doing it all alone. In fitness, in the boardroom, in baby groups, anywhere—when women come together, we can elevate one another and provide the support we all need to keep going.

TASK: IDENTIFY YOUR TRIBE

Make a list of your community, your tribe, the wonderful women (and men) in your life that you know will always have your back and you'll always have their back, too. Send them a message to say, "I've got you, I'm here for you, and we're in this together." The feeling is truly amazing.

ACCOUNTABILITY

SEVERAL TIMES A year I run a fitness challenge, anything from a seven-day to a twenty-eight-day challenge. I always tell my Tone & Sculpt familia when I'm going to start one and within a few days there are thousands of us all doing the same challenge. When I commit to one, other people do too and we all do it together. There's something about fitness challenges that massively appeals to the younger generation who are used to gaming; we all want to "win" and we feel like we've won if we complete a challenge. There's a sense of unity, fun, commitment and, of course, accountability. We share our progress with one another and we don't just celebrate every success, we keep asking and pushing to be better—as a community.

There's something about being with a friend in the gym that makes the time go faster. It's not something you should rely on—don't forget self-discipline, habit formation, routine and schedules—but working out with a friend, someone who has your back and who knows when to push you, can help you stick to those workout commitments while the habits that will last a lifetime are forming.

A while ago I posted a video of my best friend and me working out. We were in the park and I posted that we were both tired, had been working long hours and neither of us was feeling the workout at the start of it. But we showed up, we got started and we smashed it together. Why? Accountability.

We were accountable to one another and, on that day, at that time, we both needed each other to make sure we got the best out of the time we'd set aside to work out.

We both knew we wouldn't have pushed ourselves as hard if we'd trained separately because we were exhausted. But because we got together to do it, we supported each other and smashed an amazing workout together. When I was tired, we'd push for one more set and when she was tired, we'd do the same thing.

The post received several comments from people telling me that training with a buddy had made them more motivated and less likely to quit or let themselves down. That feedback most definitely made me sure I needed to include something in here about working out with a buddy.

I know we've discussed habit formation and self-discipline being the most important factors in creating a healthy lifestyle, but the more I think about it, the more I realize that a community, a buddy, can quite literally change your fitness regime as they actively make you accountable. I'd still have done the workout without my friend because I have self-discipline, but I know I wouldn't have pushed myself as hard as I did. I kept going because I felt accountable to her. If she could do one more, I could do one more. If I could do a few minutes more, so could she. We spurred each other on and had an amazing workout because of it. Accountability is a really important word and a hugely vital part of your fitness journey.

While we need to get you to a point where you don't need anyone on your path and you're accountable to yourself, at the beginning of the journey having a buddy to train with might make things easier for you. We're hardwired not to want to let other people down, which is why we're less likely to bail on a buddy than we are on ourselves.

A US study found 95 percent of participants who started a weight loss program with a friend completed the program, compared to just 76 percent who started it alone.[2] Why? Because they were accountable to one another.

Another US study looked at planking time—and we all know how tough planks can be to hold. This study had participants hold a plank on their own and then with a partner over a series of weeks. They found those who planked with a more capable partner were able to increase their plank time by 24 percent.[3] That's an awesome achievement, especially as a plank can feel never ending! Working out with a partner not only makes time fly by, it even increases your stamina. It's a win-win.

It's not just physical effort that will improve if you work out with a friend either. Studies have found those who exercise with a workout buddy are calmer after the workout than those who exercise on their own[4] and while the gym and physical exertion will release endorphins—those happy hormones you get from working out—smiling and laughing also releases those hormones and who doesn't enjoy a laugh whenever they see their friends?

You'll no doubt encourage others on the journey you're on, whether it's your kids, your friends, your work colleagues or your partner; if you know someone who's been thinking about starting their fitness journey, get them on the same page as you and embark on the journey together. While you're aiming to adopt habitual behavior, if it helps you to find a friend to work out with, do it. This is about making changes that will stay with you forever so whatever you need to get started on this path, go for it.

Try this: text your mom or your partner or your friend before you start your workout. Tell them you're starting and then tell them to text you in an hour to see if you've done it and check in to see how it went. It sounds crazy but the thought of having to send the text saying you didn't get started or decided to do something else will be enough to get you to lace up and show up. Like we've said, it's all about showing up and getting started—the rest will always follow if you can get that far.

COMPARISON SYNDROME

COMPARISON REALLY IS the thief of joy and the most frustrating thing is that we are all susceptible to it. When I started going to the gym and wanted to make training a habit, I couldn't help but look at the men and women around me and think they were better than me. I tried so hard to just focus on me, but with mirrors everywhere, I couldn't help but compare myself—my legs, my arms, my stomach! But I knew I was in the best place for me, the place that did make me happy, the place that made me feel strong and energetic and just so good about myself, especially once I got into my workout. Like with everything on your fitness journey, you must learn to overcome comparison syndrome—or at least to manage it.

There's a mistaken perception that someone else's success diminishes yours—it doesn't. I spend so much time celebrating other women and I'm pretty sure I'm happier because of it. As I explained earlier, my self-confidence comes from me and, because I truly believe in myself, I can celebrate other women's successes without feeling like their success brings shade to anything I've done or am doing.

Celebrating other women is such a huge part of what's important to me, it's what Tone & Sculpt is built upon—all succeeding, all thriving, all celebrating one another's achievements no matter how big or small. Whether you're on week one of your journey or month sixteen, you're worth celebrating and I'm here to help you do that.

Women can be so competitive—we are wracked with comparisons, always looking at how other women look, wanting what other women have, chasing the dreams of others. I can't even begin to imagine how many hours I wasted wishing I looked different from how I did, longing to look more like someone in a magazine or a movie. It's all wasted energy. The only person you should be in competition with is you— focus on your journey and make your path the best one for you. Now I look at other women in a totally different way. I admire their strength and I celebrate their authenticity.

Because that's what we all are—authentic and original. No journey or two people are the same. Never forget that.

I started doing Transformation Tuesdays forever ago. It's a platform where my followers and the Tone & Sculpt users can post their before-and-after pictures, their success stories, the fact they've changed so much since they started on their fitness journey. But, here's the thing: other women don't always like them.

It makes them question why they haven't "got there" yet. They compare themselves to what they're seeing someone else has achieved so it actually makes them feel more demotivated. I can't be in front of every single one of them but I can almost guarantee they're doing what all women do when they go to the gym—they're looking at other women around them and comparing themselves, which (as we've discussed) is utterly pointless because we're all different.

We need to change the way we look at "transformations" of women; we need to celebrate them and remember they have remained consistent and achieved their results on their own timeline—the journey is more interesting than the destination.

We should want to know more about what it took to get there, the process. We should want to know if there were tears or how hard things were. We should want to know how people coped when the going got tough, when they were tired, when they pushed themselves to work out even though the baby hadn't slept, when they thought they couldn't push themselves any more. Who supported them? How did they overcome the lulls? We should want to know it takes hard work, consistency, dedication and—always—healthy habits to make progress.

We should want to know we're not alone in the struggles. We should want to know we're not the only ones who have bad days, that we're not alone in wanting to skip a workout when we've a bad day at work. We should want to know everyone is finding it tough, that there are other people out there feeling exactly the same. The transformation photo may just show the physical change, but behind those pictures are hard work, sweat, commitment—sometimes tears, sometimes joy—that go into changing yourself and your relationship with your body and health.

You need to know the process because it will make you feel like it could be possible for you too. When you watch a cooking show on TV, do they just show you the ingredients and then the finished dish? No, because you need to know the process—it's just that cooking your favorite pasta takes a little less time than documenting a full-on fitness journey! People struggle, we all do, but knowing we're not alone when we're struggling is helpful. It keeps us going. There's a strength in the collective, and an impact when we know—as women—we're all feeling the same. People think, "If she's struggling, it's okay for me to struggle—it doesn't mean I'm doing it wrong, or that I won't get there, it just means it won't be easy and that's okay because I've seen she went through the same thing and kept going, kept showing up." That learning, that sisterhood, is so important.

Sisterhood is such a strong word. Have you ever met women you literally want to spend all your time with? Not because of how they look or what they have, but because of their *vibe*. I'm talking about the women who speak your language, understand and appreciate your outlook and have a similar drive, women who are all about being the best version of themselves. They make you feel safe, they make you feel supported and warm, and have the most infectious energy. These women draw you in because they have an inner strength; they're authentic, full of self-esteem and love for everyone around them. Those are the women you stick with, the women you surround yourself with—and be there to surround them too. That is exactly what my Tone & Sculpt ambassadors do. They are so positive and their energy and kindness is infectious. All of this comes from their fitness journeys. They sincerely and genuinely want to support one another and they are so proud of what they've all achieved—as am I! They've realized how much more fitness is and can be. Together, they've overcome issues with eating disorders and body confidence, and made friends for life. That's exactly what a community should be—friends for life.

SCULPT A COMMUNITY

"STRENGTH" AND "POWER" are two words women aren't always comfortable using but they're two of my absolute favorites and ones I want you to get used to saying and being. Strength is power. I wanted to call Tone & Sculpt "Strength" but so many people told me it's too much of a "male-orientated word." In terms of marketing, it'd be a long slog to change the way women felt about that word as it has so long been associated with being male. Well, let's hope this book can change that. Don't get me wrong, I love the name Tone & Sculpt but what a lot of people don't know is that we tone your body and we sculpt your mind so you adopt healthy habits for life. This book is the *sculpt*. You are strong, you are powerful and you can achieve anything you put your mind to. That's what all women and all children should be told every day. There are no limitations to your success and, what's more, the people in the classroom, workplace and on the train aren't in competition with you—they are there to support you.

I can take you into a gym and show you a routine that will physically change your body shape, but it's not that part of you that needs to change first. Your mind, thought process and approach to fitness is the foundation of any physical change to your body. Until we are truly confident in mind about the changes we want to make, the excuses we are willing to overcome and the habits we want to form, fitness will always just be a means to an end or a quick fix. I want my community to be running up the stairs when they're 70. I want them to be injury free throughout life. I want them to be disease free as far as possible through good health and dietary choices. And I want the movement, the pack, to keep growing, to keep getting stronger and more powerful with energy that can be embodied by women across the world.

TASK: PAY IT FORWARD

This book is for all women. I want it to help and truly empower as many women as possible (if not all women!) to work out and start their fitness journeys. I want all women to work toward becoming their best selves, for no one else but themselves. We're only halfway, but if the book is helping you, I want you to keep the message and the advice alive by sharing it with your friends, loved ones, your mom, your grandma! Let's be the best together and let's do this for all women across the world.

CHAPTER 8

EMBRACE THE FEAR

So often I hear people say to me that they're scared of weights, they're worried they're going to end up "looking like a man," they're scared about how people will look at them if they go to the gym. We need to channel that fear into performance and we need perform only for ourselves. When you learn and truly accept that you are only in this for you, you can beat that fear—trust me!

Motivational speaker Mel Robbins quite famously said fear and excitement are both real, and actually cause similar emotional reactions. The way our bodies and brains react to fear and excitement is very similar—we sweat, our hearts race, our cortisol levels go through the roof. But, like I said in Chapter 5, we need to reframe our thinking. We need to channel our nerves into excitement. If you are scared of going into the gym and starting your fitness and health journey, you need to switch it up and tell yourself, "I'm excited, I'm looking forward to the change, I can't wait to learn more about my body and be the best version of me!" See what you're doing? Straightaway your mental and emotional health is spurring you on to focus on your physical health too.

I'm terrified of swimming. I never learned when I was a child and the thought of the water petrifies me. Plus, swimming can be a hassle with getting wet, washing your hair every time…Gosh, I'm making excuses already! But, I don't want to be that person anymore. I don't want to be the one who doesn't get in the pool when I see everyone else doing it and it looks like so much fun. So, I've set myself a challenge to learn how to swim. Am I nervous? Of course! But I'm more excited by it. I can't wait to learn a new skill and I'm looking forward to seeing the amazing things it does for my mind and body. It's my own personal challenge, just for me to focus on. I don't know how to swim and I want to learn. I want to be able to get in the pool and just swim. Like I said in Chapter 7, setting challenges is fun, it's something to look forward to. Your only competition is you, it's nothing to be afraid of; instead, be excited! I dare you to try running if you haven't before, try a different sport or attempt your workouts with a barbell—you'll surprise yourself with everything you're capable of.

See what I did there? I changed my language, changed my thought process and I'm ready to beat the fear and the excuses. So what do I do next? I find a pool I can use; I either book lessons or ask a friend to swim with me for accountability (see page 87), and I make it a part of my routine by scheduling it into my calendar. Self-discipline and healthy habits will make sure swimming is something I can do by the end of next year. It's not an overnight change, but it will be a change I make, trust me.

TASK: FACE YOUR FEARS

Write down things you want to do that scare you. Write down why they scare you and then change the language to make them something you are looking forward to, like I've done with swimming. Then, write down how you're going to achieve those things. You can put down a time limit if that helps, but at this stage, writing down your action plan is an awesome way to start.

CHANGE

TO TREAD YOUR own path, especially when that path might be different from the one people think you should be on, is scary. There's a saying: *if you care about what other people think, you'll always be their prisoner.* But it's easier said than done to ignore others, especially as a woman. Society's idea of how women should be is pretty fixed. From what we achieve to who we become, women face adverse pressures, especially in the world of fitness:

- You look too "muscly."
- You're starting to look like a man.
- If you lose weight, you'll disappear!
- Are you sure you should be exercising when you're pregnant?
- Don't lift too heavy, it's not good for you!
- Women are such cardio bunnies!
- She just works out for the 'gram.

...I could go on.

I've been trolled, criticized and judged for my passion for fitness. Believe me when I say I know how hard it can be to ignore the comments, brush off the criticism and keep going. I totally understand if after a lousy day or some nasty comments, you just decide to go home and curl up with a tub of ice cream—because that's what the stereotype says. But, you are *not* a prisoner of generalizations and other people's opinions. This is why I always say you are doing this for you. Change is possible if you focus on you, and accept tunnel vision when it comes to your ambitions and your desire to change your life. No one else matters and, once you start, as soon as you put on your gym clothes or step in front of that squat rack it is only you vs. you—literally!

If you can get you to a point where you become your own inspiration, your world will change, your confidence levels will rise and you'll be as close to bulletproof as it's possible to be. The first thing to beat is the fear of change and that is something that can be accomplished through fitness. We've discussed forming healthy habits, learning new things and embracing a mindful approach to fitness. All of this is part and parcel of beating the fear of change—it's about embracing discomfort and riding with it. There's a lot of negativity in the world—you only need to look at the darker side of social media to see that. In fact, so many people avoid change and embracing new challenges because they fear "what other people may say" in the form of comments and messages on social media. You cannot give those "other people" power.

In Chapter 4, we discussed judgmental friends or partners who just don't understand your "why." You see those people frequently, you can talk to them, you can reason with them. You can make peace with the fact that they don't understand and hope that one day they will, while you continue to focus on your "why." But these mystery "keyboard ghosts" online or in the peripheries of your life? The ones who make the odd negative comment here and there? They're the ones that get to you the most! For some reason, they're the ones who affect you more than anything, yet you don't even understand why. Well let me tell you, I totally get where you're coming from, I've been there and sometimes I still find myself there. More often than I wish, I find myself wasting so much time dwelling on the few negative messages out of the hundreds that I receive. I find myself responding to them and trying to explain myself. Recently, I received a message that said it doesn't look like my back is "as strong as it was." I had no idea who this person was and maybe they were just making an observation; for them it was a fleeting comment, but for me, it hurt. I know how hard I've been training and how busy I've been with work, but it really got to me. So what did I do? I changed my training plan that day and I trained my back and upper body. It wasn't a wasted workout by any means, but it got to me to the point where I changed my plans. That is crazy!

But what's even crazier is the fear we have of those who don't even type, comment or communicate. We're scared of the ones we know or can feel are secretly judging or watching our journeys. Why are we scared? It's almost as if the fear of the unknown, the fear of imagining what people are saying is worse than any bitchy comment they throw your way. They also bring out our insecurities; perhaps we think that they are talking about the things we're uncomfortable about, the things we don't want anyone to know. It sounds irrational, but it's also completely normal.

How can we change it? How can we overcome those upsetting feelings and insecurities created by people we don't even see or know? The advice I would give you is to switch them off. Literally. If they send you negative comments, block them. If it's someone you follow, unfollow them. They only have a voice in your life when you listen to them. I know we all worry about the consequences of cutting ties, but if we're honest with ourselves we'll realize they probably won't even notice and, even if they do, they'll stop caring before tomorrow—and so should you! If you want to document your fitness journey online, why not create a separate account, a safe space for yourself? Set it to private, and only have your closest and most trusted friends on there. You then have full control over what you share and who you let into your life—just like your health and fitness journey.

You can apply similar thinking to people in real life too. We all have that friend, that neighbor or even colleague who we feel is secretly judging us, thinking about us and saying "things" about us. But, like with social media, surround yourself with people who love your energy and whose energy you love too. I know we can't always completely cut out negative people because they always somehow make an appearance, but if you train your mind, body and actions to completely immerse yourself in everything that brings you happiness, whether it's your hobbies, friends or family, you'll soon drown out the negative influences. Trust me, I've done it! Don't get me wrong, their comments play on my mind from time to time but I always think about perspective (see page 61). Are they saying anything useful? Does what they say or think have a direct impact on your life? Are their words or thoughts true? If the answer is no to these questions, then you clearly know what to do! However, if you think there is any truth in what they're saying or you know a simple conversation could iron out any awkwardness or negativity then go for it. My mom always said kindness and honesty are important, so as long as it's not hurting you in any way or bringing down your vibe, clear the air, feel confident and know that the only real opinion and judgment that matters is your own. Your gut always knows best so trust it, be confident and be with people who you trust too.

Over time, as you grow confident in your health and fitness, as you start gaining more and more control over your journey, you will learn to be your own hero. If you're your own hero, your own inspiration, none of the negative attention will affect you. You'll get to a point where you see it, you read it, but you don't *feel* it. And when you're your own inspiration, you'll never, ever let yourself down.

BE HAPPY

DON'T CONFUSE THE unknown with unhappiness. We worry about change—it's the fear of the unknown, the fear of what might be or not be. We then perceive change as something bad, hard, negative or tough—that's why changing the way you think and feel about fitness can be tough and sometimes one step forward, two steps back. It might feel right now that it's impossible for you to get to a place where you see fitness and strength the way I do—as something that's second nature and as ingrained into my day as brushing my teeth—but trust me, it will happen and it will happen in a way that suits you and your happiness.

I knew being fit and healthy would make me happy but my version was obsessing over the scale, constantly counting calories and only eating brown rice, broccoli and chicken—and I was tired of it. I started moving away from that and, while I didn't know I was heading to a lifelong relationship with strength training, it interested me and I started to enjoy training so much more. It doesn't matter what kind of training you choose, you just need to make sure it's something that makes you happy, something that you look forward to and enjoy.

At work so many of us have performance reviews. For some reason, many of us grow scared of them; we worry about how well we're doing, whether we've met our targets or even if we're going to keep the job we're in! Why do we always jump to the negative? I guess it's human nature, it's where our fight-or-flight instinct sometimes kicks in, where our brain jumps to our defense and into protection mode when we fear something. Women have a tendency to reflect on the negative more than the positive—we are definitely "glass half empty." We want to tick ALL the boxes before we go for a promotion, whereas men go for it even if they only tick three! We end up feeling frustrated, restless and, basically, unhappy. We need to be more "glass half full" and we need to apply positive and confident thinking to our training too. When we look in the mirror, we need to see and believe everything we've achieved instead of focusing on negative thoughts. Stop staring at your butt thinking it's not the right shape (what even is the right shape?); stop finding faults with your body and instead focus on the fact that you're in your gym gear, you're about to smash it in the gym or you've just completed your best session yet—and that is something to be super-proud of.

BE GRATEFUL

LIKE WE DID in Chapter 5, let's reframe our thinking around training to make us happy and grateful for what our bodies can achieve:

- I want to make time to exercise because it's time for me; it's important to me and it makes me happy.
- I will end my workout feeling energized, refreshed and ready to get on with my day.
- The days I get to work out and complete my workout are my best days.
- My workouts fit comfortably into my schedule and I look forward to them.

Embrace your workouts and know they are there to make you happy, not scare you. Each workout and exercise routine is fulfilling. You're gaining and learning so much, and you need to be grateful for what your body can do for you. Workouts are there to protect us, to energize us, to enable us to take care of ourselves, our friends and our families.

Fear has a funny way of taking over and can affect the gray matter in our brains. In fact, there is a link between the gray matter and exercise. Our brain's cerebrum is rich with gray matter, which contains countless neuronal cell bodies. The cerebrum is the part that is responsible for conscious movement, our emotions, how we see, feel and process things, and even how we make decisions. The cerebrum, forming the outer regions of the brain, helps to manage how we process information, especially events and experiences that affect our emotions. Research suggests that, as we get older, our gray matter shrinks. Perhaps this is why the more basal "fight or flight" instinct is more likely to kick in, and we are more likely to get stressed and let feelings like fear take over.

Meditation and mindfulness can help strengthen and even increase the gray matter in your brain and can reduce signs of aging.[1] This is where exercise can make a difference. Exercise can be a form of mindfulness, a time to zone out and focus on just you. It can calm your stress levels, release endorphins and make you feel great! It can help you practice gratitude and make you thankful for the small things, the small wins throughout your day:

- I managed a twenty-minute workout today and have so much more energy because of it.
- I am so grateful for my body; I managed to squat an extra 10 lbs. today and felt so strong.
- My back pain is slowly disappearing and my core feels so much stronger from the ab workouts I've been doing.
- I exercised outside today and soaked up the sunshine.
- I had to change around my schedule this week but still managed to do all my workouts.
- I tried a new healthy recipe and it was super-tasty!
- My friend and I tried a new spin class—I'm so grateful to have a gym buddy.

We shouldn't be scared of fitness and the journey. Instead, we should be grateful for the opportunity to do better, feel great and be our best!

TASK: RECORD YOUR ACHIEVEMENTS

Take pride in everything you've achieved, from picking up this book to smashing your most recent workout. After each workout, keep a note of one thing that you feel good about after your workout session. What made you feel proud today? Do this after every workout and, trust me, you won't want to miss a single one!

I've had enough experience to know that when I have seismic shifts in my life, I stop and try my best to learn from them and make changes, however big or small, in reaction to them. Maybe moving countries, learning a new language and integrating into a different culture helped with that—whatever it may be, change doesn't need to be scary, it just makes you more resilient and helps you identify with yourself more.

No matter how I dress it up, the plain and simple fact is that being uncomfortable and facing your fears leads to change and growth; even if you find out the change isn't for you, it's still growth. You've learned something about yourself, something that's only going to make future decisions more confident and more accurate.

Change is no more a threat than it is an opportunity, an opportunity to learn more about yourself, to love yourself that little bit more and to do more for you too.

CHAPTER 9

BE MORE THAN MOTIVATED

I f you have to rely on motivation and willpower, if they're what get you out the door and into the gym, you might be making your journey harder than it needs to be. Let me start by saying motivation is fake. That phrase, "you've got to find the motivation," is totally misleading, false and begs the question, "Where?" It's the same as saying, "You've got to find the willpower." Oh, and my favorite, "Be resilient."

If you've ever been given a motivational speech at school, at work or even online that fires you up for the day, but then find you're back to square one, ask yourself why. What's missing? I mean, to be fair, someone might say this entire book is motivating. It may well be, but I'd argue that motivation is just a short-term side effect of the content and is by no means the reason you should pick it up. In fact, I'd be disappointed in myself if you saw it as motivating and nothing else. The reason is that, yes, I want you to read this book; yes, I want it to make you feel good; I want you to know I am here for you, but the book is a waste of your money if you don't treat it like your action plan. There is a reason for all the tasks and why I keep mentioning habits, self-discipline, consistency and routine.

If you believe someone is motivated to achieve success, or you think someone is successful because they are motivated, you're wrong. What they are is disciplined, focused and they take action. THEN motivation may come, when they realize their habits and consistency are making them successful. So what do they do? They don't "stay motivated," they just stick to their habitual behavior and their routine. And, if they realize something isn't working, they don't just stop—they change habits, they try something new and keep going. It's not motivation that keeps people going, it's routine and habits.

The same applies to your fitness and health journey. It's like sweets vs. a balanced meal: sweets give you a quick sugar rush and a bit of energy and sometimes that's all you need. But for long-lasting energy you need a balanced meal to keep you going for a number of hours and to sustain a healthy lifestyle. It's the healthy meals and consistent fitness routine that you need to keep going—not just a one-off, instant rush. Build the habits, stay consistent and keep trying different things until you learn what works for you. Discipline and focus need to come before feelings of motivation. With focus and discipline, you will build healthy habits, and healthy habits will breed feelings of resilience.

THE MYTH OF MOTIVATION

MOTIVATION IN A broader context is linked to your "why"—your passion, purpose and reasons are the motivation that drives you. But looking motivation it in isolation and hoping it'll be enough to get you to lace up your tennis shoes and get going is a dangerous path to be on. Daily motivation comes and goes and at times even your "why" can be blurred. What happens if you injure yourself? Move house? Change jobs? Have a baby? Even if these don't apply to you, you can empathize with the feelings of resilience and motivation fading a little. Motivation comes and goes, resilience changes too—you can't rely on them, it's just not sustainable. In fact, sometimes I wonder whether motivation becoming a buzzword is what leaves people feeling so lost and unmotivated. I'm no doctor or specialist, but if we're constantly being told to "stay motivated" without knowing how or why to "stay motivated," no wonder so many of us feel deflated a lot of the time! So for me, it becomes a myth; we know it's meant to be something amazing and life changing, but we just don't really understand the truth of it.

GOOD DAYS AND BAD DAYS

EVERYONE HAS THOSE days when they feel like they can take on the world and win—the house or apartment is cleaned top to bottom in the morning; the laundry basket is emptied; the dinner is prepped early. We all know those days when we accomplish loads that wasn't on our list because we think our motivation levels are so high—we're winning at life! On the flipside, though, we also recognize those days when even the bare minimum is an effort. The days when the sofa beckons all day long and all you want to do is binge-watch your favorite shows on Netflix and spend the day on social media. Those are the days when you feel motivation has deserted you—you can't find it, you kind of don't want to or can't be bothered anyway. Like the weather, sometimes it's on your side and you're loving life, sometimes it's not and all you do is cancel plans and curl up indoors.

Although you can't control the weather, you shouldn't let it interrupt your schedule, just as you shouldn't let a lack of motivation on any given day derail your routine. Yes, you may need to adapt (change the gym session to a home workout, train for thirty minutes instead of sixty), but if you maintain control over your healthy habits and thought process, no given mood can control you—you control it! If you need a TV day, have a TV day, just make sure you're the one who is in control, be mindful that we all need rest, we all need kindness and that too comes with self-discipline. Although, as your trainer, I have to say that even a rest day can involve a few stretches in front of the TV or a nice walk after dinner. Plus, you don't need to consume a whole tub of ice cream in one sitting—be mindful and eat a few scoops instead (more on food to come later).

CAN I RELY ON MOTIVATION?

DON'T GET ME wrong, I know I said that motivation is fake. But equally, I know it's a real feeling too. To feel motivated and unmotivated is real. But, it's not something you can rely on, which is why I have a problem with the phrase "find motivation" to make things work. I see motivation as an add-on. It's like a supplement. Supplements shouldn't be relied on and in the same way you shouldn't rely on motivation. Supplements are exactly that; they're meant to supplement the diet you already have, which should be a good, healthy and balanced one.

There's no point taking supplements if your diet and workouts aren't good and it's the same with motivation. It won't do its job if you don't have organized, structured habits. That's why scheduling and routine are so important—and I know I keep coming back to them, but they are the backbone to achieving your goals.

I also find motivation has a cycle. It's easy to be motivated at the start of the week when you've got a spring in your step and you've had a good weekend. But, if you get to the end of Monday and it's been an intense day in the office with a few stressful meetings, you'll feel super-unmotivated and even likely to skip the gym. By the end of the week, your motivation levels have dropped, you're longing for the weekend and you don't think twice about ditching a workout for a glass of wine with colleagues after work or the sofa and your favorite series.

Then when Saturday morning comes around and your alarm goes off—despite the fact that you laid out your clothes last night, charged your headphones and got your plan and fitness tracker ready—you press the snooze button and have a nice long sleep. Before you know it, it's time for brunch or an appointment, and your workout is a distant memory. You're not alone—we've all been there—but that's a classic example of your motivation deserting you. You went to sleep relying on the fact your motivation would get you up in the morning and it's disappeared overnight.

Not only that but there's the very real possibility you'll spend the rest of the day feeling guilty and you'll spend hours trying to find a window of time you can fit it in. In short, your day won't be as good as it would have been if you'd stuck to your commitment to get up, smash a workout, forget about it and get on with your day.

However, if you've built the habit, you'll be up and at the gym without a second thought. You've planned that Saturday-morning workout, you scheduled it last week, you value yourself and the commitment you made to yourself so it doesn't even enter your head not to follow through with what you've planned. In short, you have discipline. Discipline and consistency trump motivation every day of the week.

I promise you, relying on the habit and having it scheduled will give you so much more headspace because it's hardwired into you, it's second nature and it's almost like a reflex.

DISCIPLINE

I KNOW I'M ASKING you to change a lot about yourself through this book, but one of the most important things I can ask of you is that you don't rely on motivation. Rely on discipline.

Discipline is unending. It's stability, it's structure, it's unwavering. Forget motivation that—like the moon—will be full and bright on occasion only to dim and slim through the passage of the day or the month. Discipline won't ever fail you. Ever.

WILLPOWER

A US STUDY SEPARATED participants into two groups—both were told not to eat anything for three hours before the study.[1] One group was placed in a room with a plate of chocolate chip cookies, the other placed in a room with radishes. The radish group were told they could eat as many radishes as they wanted but the cookie group were asked not to eat the cookies. After a few hours, both groups were given a puzzle to solve but they didn't know the puzzle was impossible. The group who had used their willpower to resist eating the cookies gave up on the puzzle far faster than those who'd been in the room with the radishes. It showed what scientists have suspected for years, that willpower is unreliable and isn't always there when you need it, especially if you've already exhausted it on resisting something else.

Willpower can only get you so far if you're not organized. I've had times when I've had so much willpower, but I haven't organized when I'll work out or got my gym gear ready and then the day gets away from me or I realize my gear is in the wash or I can't find my tracker or resistance bands…and then the willpower disappears and I get frustrated.

A lot of people will tell you that willpower is the key to their success, that it made them get up earlier, write the book faster, stick to their commitments, or climb up the ladder of promotions. Either they're not telling you the full truth or they're not giving themselves enough credit. Like motivation, willpower is also an add-on; if you build good habits and organize your time and priorities, willpower will be there to spur you on. Without habits, routine and discipline, willpower is just a nice word. Being effective and organized are what you want to focus your energy on, not willpower. If you approach the lessons in this book the right way and form the habits you can hardwire and rely on, you won't need willpower. Fitness will become an intrinsic part of your life and you'll celebrate the lifestyle it gives you. I don't always have willpower but I always have the discipline to be consistent. It's the same discipline that helped me work hard for and pass my law degree; it's the same discipline that got me on time for every shift at work no matter how exhausted I was when I was waitressing. That discipline started Tone & Sculpt and grew it into the business it is today—with discipline anything is possible.

Willpower is not an unrelenting, perpetually stocked bank you can keep drawing on. So if you've had to exercise willpower not to bite back at a snarky colleague in a meeting, or had to concentrate and pay attention at work all morning, you're less likely to have enough left in reserve to get you into the gym at the end of a busy day. However, like a muscle, willpower can be worked and made stronger and bigger—with the help of healthy habits and discipline. From being patient with annoying colleagues to avoiding the second or third piece of cake at a birthday party, relying solely on willpower can be exhausting. So, for things like your spin class or legs session, I urge you to rely on your schedule and routine instead.

RESILIENCE

RESILIENCE COMES FROM our experiences, our learning and from the understanding of those experiences and the outcomes of them. It's one of those character traits we'd all like to think we have, and we'd be pleased if someone else described us as being resilient. It's of such importance that the World Health Organization has identified building resilience as a "key pillar" of its framework for improving health and well-being. People say that being resilient means you are "strong." For me, resilience has more to do with how you manage difficult times and what things you can rely on to help you get through them.

But here's the thing: resilience is a variable and it's not something we have a huge amount of control over because it can be situation-based. For example, if you change jobs, lose a loved one, gain a loved one, move house or country, meet new friends—all of this can affect your resilience, which can then affect your routines and habits if you are relying on it. Resilience, in my experience, depends on how you react to different situations. We've discussed the fear of change and fight-or-flight instinct, and it's these feelings and reactions that affect our resilience. Some people have their resilience tested daily and some very rarely.

The amount of change I've experienced since childhood has really tested my resilience. From moving countries, learning a new language, starting classes, to nearly being homeless, it's been tough. And anyone close to me will know the greatest challenge for me was ending my engagement with my fiancé, best friend and business partner, Jack. I cannot tell you how tough that was. I felt completely broken. I went between knowing it was the right decision for both of us, to regret, panic and hating myself. It was awful. I didn't really know what to do or who I was. But, after letting myself grieve (and of course my routine went out of the window for a while), I got back to it. I spent time with myself, I got back into training, eating right and eventually (and I'll always be working on it) things started to fall into place again. I remembered my "why," my vision, my purpose and reasons—and all of that came back to me once my routine and self-discipline were back in action. I guess that's what resilience is: you have to take control of your life to be and feel confident, motivated and resilient.

Mindset and how we view adversity and hardship has a lot to do with our motivation, willpower and resilience. Think about when you see people on the news who have survived something terrible—a plane crash or a house fire. There'll be some who say their lives are over, that it's the worst thing that's happened to them—and arguably it is. But there'll be others who say they're so lucky to have survived, that they feel blessed to have made it out. Resilience—in part—is also about how you frame things. Think back to Chapter 5 on perspective: if you've had a run of bad luck and things have been going wrong, you have two options. You can look at it as a run of bad luck and feel like you're never going to get a break, that all the bad luck happens to you. Or you can think of solutions to fix everything that's happened. Whichever outcome or feeling you go with will determine and test your level of resilience. In scenario one, you won't have much resilience because you'll feel like you've been a bit beaten by things. Whereas in scenario two, you'll feel like you've weathered a bad week and you're on to new things—you survived what was thrown at you and are better and stronger for it.

Resilience can be built over time and studies have found that exercise can boost resilience in other areas of your life, from work to relationships. But, it's a "boost"—at the foundation is still the workout, the habits, the routine and the consistency. Nothing can replace discipline, organization, commitment, scheduling, habits and consistency. Let's say it again: be consistent, have a routine and form healthy habits.

WHERE DOES MY MOTIVATION COME FROM?

I SPEND EVERY SUNDAY or Monday morning working out my routine for the week in terms of fitness. I decide what I'm going to do and when I'm going to do it. I write down my workouts or I use the Tone & Sculpt app to choose and schedule them. I usually take time out on a Sunday to meal prep and plan. This might include a supermarket visit, batch cooking and making sure there is enough to keep me going throughout the week. While I'm doing this, I also look at my work and meeting schedule, as this will obviously have an impact on my eating plans. All of the above are habits. It is a routine. I feel motivated after I've done this as it liberates me. It gives me free time to think—my schedule is set in stone, I know exactly what I'm doing, when I'm doing it and now I can think about all of the other time I have to chill, read a book or spend time with loved ones. My life literally is *that* exciting!

What do I do if something gets in the way? We said life happens and obviously not every day is going to be perfect or exactly how you planned it. But this is where you refer back to perspective and mindset: be flexible and kind to yourself and try to do the next best thing. For example, for me, if something goes wrong at work, or an unexpected meeting comes up—which happens often when you're starting a business—I have to adapt. I'll take a look at my schedule and just shift a few things around. Because my schedule and routine are already there, I don't need to panic; I just visually make it all work another way. Panic over. You can always have control of the situation. Equally, I try to always make sure my environment is set up to suit my schedule and routine too—I'm nearly always wearing a sports bra so I can always work out! I wear my gym clothes or keep them with me so I'm ready for a workout. I set up my workout space at home beforehand so there are literally no excuses. Do your best to remove the obstacles and just get on with it. The more you think about working out, the more time you'll waste—just get it in your schedule and get on with it!

My motivation comes from having the headspace to focus

on other things, as my workouts and meal planning are hard-wired into my calendar, so I don't have to think about them. I don't need willpower, resilience or motivation because the workouts are habits I've formed and I wouldn't dream of letting myself down. I'm disciplined and nothing is getting in the way of that. Just remember, this type of thinking and mindset takes time. It needs to be nurtured, you need to prioritize yourself and take the time to focus on you. It's the only way to really do this for you.

NOTHING'S WORKING

OKAY, LET'S BE real. There will be times when you feel habits, routine, motivation—just about everything—is letting you down. You feel trapped, you've hit a wall and you have no idea how to get through it or walk away from it. I've been there too. We need to think back to mindful fitness and reflecting. We need to remember we're on a journey, and it's not a race where you just keep looking forward. Remember what I said: you have to look back to move forward. Here are a few questions to ask yourself when you have hit a wall:

- Have you changed the time you're working out?
- Have you switched up your diet or have you changed your eating pattern?
- What did you eat before you came to work out?
- Are you sleeping well? How many hours of sleep are you getting a night?
- Is it your time of the month?
- Have you just finished a busy project at work?

- Are you getting along with your friends and family? No dramas?
- Have you managed to socialize with people recently?

As well as having a "why" to inspire us to keep going, we need to question ourselves about what might be holding us back, too. So many things in life can have an impact on our training schedules and it's important that we're mindful of them so we know how to utilize the positives and overcome the negatives. When you come up with an answer and then a solution, you'll be ready to adapt your schedule and get back at it!

TASK: REFLECT ON YOUR MOTIVATION

Try to think of a time when your motivation, willpower and resilience have let you down. It could be something as big as changing jobs and not feeling motivated by it, or always going for that second or third doughnut and then feeling really guilty. Now think why. Make a list of reasons why you felt let down and what you could have done to change that. For example, with the job, is it because it's a new environment, you don't feel comfortable with the change, there is stuff you need to learn? If so, how can you make it comfortable, and what habits and routines can you put in place to feel confident in it?

Whatever way you look at it, this task can really help you reflect and overcome challenging feelings about lack of motivation and resilience. Remember, there is always a solution, it just takes time and patience.

CHAPTER 10

BUILD YOUR STRENGTH

Anthropologically, men are considered to be the hunters, while women are the gatherers. We're called "the weaker sex" or "the second sex." I've said it before that strength and power are words not usually associated with femininity and even though that's slowly changing, celebration of strong women is still so rare. Michelle Obama, Jacinda Ardern, Beyoncé, Serena Williams...all of these women are strong and powerful, but there are many more male figureheads we can name. Being female and strong goes against the grain of what we've been taught to believe for centuries, no matter what culture, religion or planet you're from. But it's changing. Slowly but surely it's changing, with women like you, me and so many others ready to shift the status quo, so that women can be seen as strong, not just in the gym but in life in general, standing on our own with no comparison to any male counterpart.

Get ready for a long chapter, one where I'm going to teach you as much as I can about strength training to the point where you'll be joining me with your dumbbells in hand very, very soon.

MEN VS. WOMEN

WE ALL CONSTANTLY have glossy magazines and Hollywood idols to compare ourselves with. When I joined the gym, I had a vision of what I wanted to look like and I didn't think I looked like it. I didn't look like the women I saw on TV or in the media that I wanted to emulate, and rather than looking in the mirror and seeing what I was or the positive things about myself, I'd look at my reflection and see all the things I wasn't. Like so many women I know, I spent my teens feeling really insecure about myself. I'd spend hours looking at my reflection, wishing it was different; noticing that a feature of mine was smaller or bigger than it "should be."

When I joined the gym and started training, it was in part because I wanted a curvier physique. But within a few weeks, that gave way to wanting to be strong. I saw physical strength in the other people in the gym, particularly men, and I wanted a slice of that. I focused on a physical goal in those first few weeks I was training but, within a really short period of time, I changed that aesthetic ideal for a mindful one. Strength was what I wanted. I loved pushing myself and the thought of being stronger, and therefore able to do more, was so appealing it changed my whole reason for being there. I ditched the idea of a metric, a measurement or a number on the scale, and went for strength instead. It didn't take long for me to shift my goal from an aesthetic one to one that would serve me for the rest of my life, the same goal I have today: to grow stronger and more advanced every time, every session.

There's a massive confidence gap between the genders, but I only really noticed it when I joined a gym. Men would stroll into the weights section far more confidently than women, who could look so self-conscious and vulnerable. With every visit I realized I wanted to narrow the gap between male and female strength; I wanted them to be on a par with one another. Neither one should be "better" than the other, but everyone should just want to be the best they can be.

Why? Why didn't women feel as confident in this environment as men did? Why did men treat the strength section of the gym like their second home, but women would walk past it without making eye contact like they were avoiding a long-lost ex? Why did men seem to warm up by the bench and take full control of the weights for an hour or so, but women would spend their entire workout not leaving the vicinity of the treadmill? Now, don't get me wrong, there is absolutely nothing wrong with a treadmill, cross trainer or whatever piece of equipment so long as you *enjoy* it and *want* to train with it. However, I have a big problem if a woman feels she *can't* use a particular piece of equipment because it's not for her. That's simply *not true*.

WHY STRENGTH TRAIN?

SO MANY WOMEN say to me they don't want to strength train because:

- They don't want big muscles.
- They "only" want to tone.
- They worry they might hurt themselves.
- They're not strong enough.
- And, my personal favorite, they don't want to look like a man!

Seriously, none of the above is accurate. Strength training may not be our default setting (because, let's be honest, it's always been promoted as a man thing) but strength training has so many benefits for women:[1]

You will lose body fat

Studies show that it is not simply cardio exercises or HIIT training that helps with weight loss. Strength training can help increase your lean muscle and reduce your body fat. When we think weights make us "bulky" it's not true. Excess body fat does. So many women are concerned with losing "weight" when the focus should be "body fat." Put simply, your focus should be a healthy, balanced lifestyle, and if you need to reduce your body fat, you need to be mindful of your energy (calorie) consumption and you need to incorporate strength training.

You will gain strength

Strength is important. You need to feel like you can lift that box, climb the ladder and carry the shopping all the way up three flights of stairs. You want to be able to throw your children, grandchildren, nieces and nephews up in the air (albeit, safely!). You want to be crawling around with them or taking your dog for long walks without being out of breath. Strength training is liberating for every part of your lifestyle, physically and mentally.

You will see an improvement in back pain and posture

As strength training needs you to engage your key muscles and joints, it is an extremely beneficial way of supporting your back and core and improving your posture. When our muscles are weak, we feel weak, so strengthening them is the key to minimizing pain and stiffness, and increasing bone density, as we grow old. For women in particular, strength training is also a great preventative measure for osteoporosis.

You reduce the risk of disease

You may have heard of visceral fat—this is the type of fat that surrounds your internal organs. You can be any shape or size, but your organs could be telling a different story. A combination of strength training and aerobic training can prevent the regaining of visceral fat.[2] Heart disease, diabetes, high blood pressure—the risk of all of these can be reduced with strength training. Resistance-based exercises support your bones and joints and strengthen your muscles to ensure your body is functioning healthily and optimally. Remember, strength training also challenges your cardiovascular system (trust me, you can get as much of a sweat on at the squat bar as you can running 5k). And don't forget, your heart is a muscle too. By strengthening all of your key muscles, you are putting yourself in better health.

You reduce feelings of anxiety, stress and depression

A US study found the greatest benefits to mental health came when participants lifted moderate weights at about 70 percent of their maximum capacity.[3] I am living proof that lifting and strength training make you happier and healthier. The energy and endorphins released during a resistance-based workout are so good for you. Strength training leaves you ready to face and conquer the world in a way I never thought was possible. You push yourself, you focus and you succeed to the point where you enjoy the muscle burn and you welcome the DOMS (delayed onset muscle soreness) the next day! It leaves you feeling strong and able to manage and overcome negative feelings.

Being strong and powerful in fitness or in the gym will build feelings of resilience, which you'll carry into every other part of your life. When you push yourself in a workout, you start to realize you can advocate for yourself in other areas of your life. Think about it, we usually aim to push ourselves to "failure" when we're working out. We say, "just one more rep," or "just one more minute." And, by the end, we realize we've done it, we won. Strength training helps you feel and be more ambitious in the things you take on because you won't be as scared of failure.

But I'll end up looking like a man

This one gets me. Every. Single. Time. I've been training for years now and let me tell you something: you just get stronger, fitter, leaner, better. That is all! We are not built like men. We don't have the same level of testosterone for our muscles to grow in a similar way to men. Instead, we tone, we sculpt, we get strong. Muscle definition will come, but you also have to watch your diet. Ultimately, if you want to put on size, you're going to need to eat more, especially protein. If that's what you would like to work toward, fine (but like I've said, remember your primary "why" more than anything). But as long as you're eating a consistently healthy, balanced diet, you have nothing to worry about. You will always look like you and that's the best way to be!

But it's not pretty

I'm sorry, what? So many women tell me they can't train hard, because it's not pretty. They don't like the way they look when they scrunch up their face as they squat. They go too red. They sweat too much. They smell. I have a really big issue with femininity and fitness. Being strong, working hard and pushing new limits are just not associated with being feminine. Ask yourself whether you'd ever bat an eyelid at a man sweating in the gym? Would you ever question a man for screwing up his face because he was so intensely focusing on his progress? Would you ever judge a man for trying to catch his breath because he's just achieved his personal best in his deadlift? We need to normalize strength, power, determination and discipline for women too—it *is* feminine, it's attractive and it's everything a woman should be.

We need to stop focusing on aesthetics. I know you want to look good, I know you have a particular image in mind, but focusing just on aesthetics is a barrier to true strength and inner confidence. It is temporary. The feeling of "looking good" is not sustainable as it is constantly changing and ever-evolving. It's a marketing tactic and one that's pretty powerful as it's working on you right now. Well, let's break it. Now.

The gym isn't a fashion show: it's a place to get physically stronger and better. You come in, you train and you leave. You might grab a coffee or a shake on the way out, but then you leave and you get on with your day. That's what it is, that's all it is. If you're viewing it as anything else, you are trying to make it something it isn't. Training, whether it is cardio or strength, is a tool for you to be the best version of yourself. Think back to the first few chapters—we discussed mindset and shifting our thinking patterns. Always remember training is about how it makes you feel, the difference it makes to your life internally. If you keep chasing a particular image that you don't see in the mirror, you won't ever be happy and you won't ever be doing this for you—you're simply doing it for a quick fix, compliment, picture or pair of jeans and that is not sustainable.

You need sustainability in your workouts. You need to keep going for life, not just until you reach the physical goal or the number on the scale or the tape measure. You've already learned why it's important you keep working out for life, what a difference fitness at every age can make, so if you're in your twenties or thirties, think about what you'll feel like if you're still chasing a smaller waist or a curvier booty when you're in your fifties. How tiring that'll be to have your happiness and confidence determined by a scale or a dress size. Health and wellness should be your goal and that's something you can work at and embody throughout life.

STRENGTH AND SELF-ESTEEM

THE DEFINITION OF self-esteem is "confidence in one's own worth or abilities." I think there is a slight difference between confidence and self-esteem. We've already discussed confidence and, in my opinion, although confidence is rooted in self-esteem, sometimes we can be "confident" in all that we have achieved, see and do, but we don't necessarily *feel it*. Like my mom always says, you have to be strong *inside*, meaning your self-esteem must always, always come from you. You have to be your own inspiration, your own best friend, your own sense of strength. If your self-esteem comes from someone else's compliments, a good pair of jeans or a simple reflection in the mirror, it's probably in a delicate balance and could be tilted pretty easily. When it comes from places other than you, it's fragile in its existence and can disappear.

Think about it for a second: if you get self-esteem by the number on the scale, if that changes then your self-esteem plummets. If it comes from someone else complimenting you, when those compliments disappear or don't come for whatever reason, you start wondering if you're enough. If it comes from fitting into a certain pair of jeans or a dress, the second you can't, your whole day is ruined and you feel bad about yourself. Where self-esteem comes from is as important as the feeling itself.

When self-esteem comes from what you can do, rather than how you're perceived, that's when it's infallible. People can say what they like about me but I know I'm strong, I know what I can lift and what I can do and how my body can push itself, and that's not something anyone can affect—that's where my confidence is rooted and it's pretty unwavering. My self-esteem comes from me, no one else, and not only am I pretty bulletproof because of that, but I know the person who gives me that self-esteem isn't going anywhere. They're not going to change their mind or turn against me because it's me. I'm my own cheerleader.

Of course I have bad days, days when I feel lousy, but that's where mindful fitness, habitual behavior and self-discipline come into play; I refocus, I train and my self-esteem is right there with me.

When I feel strong and powerful, I feel like nothing can stop me, that I can take anything on and succeed. I feel like that after those sessions in the gym when I'm dripping with sweat and have pushed myself harder than I thought possible.

When I'm out of breath and I'm in the zone pushing it, I feel incredible—that's when I feel I'm at my best. When my legs are shaking, when my heart is pounding, when I'm so focused on finishing the movement I'm in, I feel confident. When I don't care who is in front of me, or what people are thinking of me, that's when my self-esteem is high. That moment in the zone when it's just me—me and my strength and that's all I'm focusing on and all I'm thinking about—that's when I feel amazing, powerful and like I could take on anything in life.

Working out is where I obtain my self-confidence and self-esteem, my power and strength and ability to smash a challenge I wasn't sure I could when I started.

Achievement, success, strength, power—for me those are all the words I associate with being female, confident and amazing. What I can do means far more to me than what I look like.

HOW DO I STRENGTH TRAIN?

S o YOU NOW know *why* you should be strength training and the health benefits it'll give you inside and out, but what actually is it? Strength training isn't just about barbells, dumbbells and repetitive lifting. It's about understanding *how* it can fit into your fitness routine and *what* you need to consider.

Form

Form is about how you actually do the exercises themselves, how you hold the dumbbell, how you plank, how you hold your body when you're doing a push-up or a bicycle crunch.

It can also involve your breathwork—when do you inhale and when do you exhale?

Having the correct form will not only increase the effectiveness of your workout, so that you're working the muscle groups you're targeting properly and maximizing every movement, but it will also prevent injury. Planking with your butt in the air won't do your core as much good than if you're holding the plank correctly with back, neck, shoulders and butt in line. Likewise, when you are performing squats, make sure your knees are in line with your toes and not rotated inward to prevent you from putting unnecessary strain on your knee joints. It's not worth cheating on form because you won't get out of it what you're putting in and you could leave yourself prone to injury. If anything, just do one less rep if you are feeling fatigued.

If you're not on the Tone & Sculpt app already (I know I'm biased), that's where you'll find all the tutorials on form you need. There are also plenty of online resources that will show you the correct way to perform every exercise—all just an internet search away.

Technique

Once you have perfected your form, it's time to move on to technique. For many strength-training exercises, you can vary the technique. It's the small incremental ways you can challenge yourself, add some variety to your routine and level up. For example, when you're bench pressing, that's the form. The technique of bench pressing can be done with a close grip or a wide grip—it's the same exercise and the same form but the different grip techniques will work different muscles in your chest. You'll find some techniques hard and some more manageable. You might also find, depending on your mobility and range of movement, some techniques work for you and some might not.

However, your technique should constantly evolve and change so that you're getting an all-over workout and changing things up every few weeks. Otherwise you risk getting bored of your routine or overworking the same muscle group. Technique allows you to spend longer with the same piece of equipment but get so much more than one exercise out of it. The same equipment with different techniques can work tons of different muscle groups.

Bodyweight training

Some might argue this isn't the same thing as strength training, but I believe utilizing your own body weight to build strength is one of the simplest and easiest ways to strength train. When I don't have time to go to the gym or I have limited equipment to use, using my own body weight and resistance to train is perfect. While I do use weights a lot when I work out, I love the fact I don't need anything other than myself and my own body to do a strength-training program. By training with my own body weight, I am effectively learning to lift and control myself. If you travel for work, all you need is yourself and some space in your hotel room to work out, so there really are no excuses. Think:

- Push-ups
- Tricep dips
- Planks
- Squats
- Lunges

The beauty of strength training is that it doesn't need to be overcomplicated. The exercises above can be done with or without weights. I would highly recommend you experiment with these exercises at home or at a gym. Consult a personal trainer or gym instructor for in-person advice or take a look at the Tone & Sculpt app and social media channels—there are tutorials for each and every one of these exercises.

Weights, reps and sets

Weights: how many kilograms or pounds you are lifting.

Reps: stands for "repetitions," so the number of times you repeat a particular exercise or movement. Aim for anything between eight to fifteen repetitions of each exercise, depending on the level of weight you are lifting.

Sets: the number of rounds of reps you complete for a particular exercise. Aim for three sets and build your way up to five.

Weights, reps and sets are important because they help you time and plan your workouts effectively and efficiently. You may think you need to do several squats and lunges, but without knowing what weight or how many you're doing, you may walk away from a workout unaware of how effective you've been.

Typically, as a rule of thumb, try the following:

Light weight: you could rep those squats out for a good few minutes without breaking a sweat or needing to catch your breath.

Moderate weight: you can feel your muscles engage and some tension by the time you repeat twelve to fifteen repetitions.

Heavy weight: you cannot hold a conversation while repping it out and can just about manage eight to ten repetitions.

> ### TASK: STAND UP AND GET MOVING
>
> Make sure you move every day. Why not set an alert on your phone to remind you to do ten push-ups every couple of hours? Or to prompt you to get up from your desk and go for a walk around the office, around the garden, or even up and down the stairs? Movement, no matter what it is, is good for you, so get up, get moving and enjoy it!

Endurance

This is one of the most challenging but rewarding parts of strength training to crack. Strength training is a skill and learning new skills is meant to be difficult. You persevere, you endure and that's how you learn. Often, the more you learn a new skill, the easier it gets; however, it's the opposite with strength training. As you master the skills of form, technique and the different types of exercises, strength training gets harder and more challenging because that's how you progress. I've done plenty of different sports and exercises in my life and nothing builds endurance—mentally and physically—like strength training. When you get to that magic point when you can endure a workout that seemed like a pipe dream a month ago, you'll feel so proud of yourself—that feeling of being strong and successful is addictive, trust me. At that point, you challenge yourself even more; you increase the weight, reps and sets depending on what you want to achieve and that's how you learn to get better and better. You might change up your routine too. Either way, you've got to endure the challenge to enjoy the reward.

Performance

Your performance will improve as long as you are consistent with your workouts. You won't feel *as* exhausted as you did at the start of your journey, your movements will be cleaner and slicker and you'll be more confident in yourself as your performance improves. I know several personal trainers say it doesn't matter what you do, as long as you move. This is a hundred percent true. However, there will come a point when you will want to add that extra challenge, you will want to "upskill" in your fitness. Improving your performance can help with this. Over time, you'll have fewer "off" days, fewer times when you don't feel you did as well as you could have done. Consistency is vital for good performance, which is why habits and routine are so important. I never switch up a gym program unless I've done it for over a month. There are so many different things you can do, but jumping around every session and never having the same routine won't give you time to see changes. I stick to the same workout for four to five weeks and then I change it. But when I change it, I don't always start doing something completely different. I sometimes keep the same routine but add in new principles, such as these:

Time Under Tension (TUT) will massively intensify your workouts. It's the amount of time a muscle is held in the "strain phase." So, if you're performing a simple curl with a dumbbell, you hold the movement at the toughest point—when you feel the muscles engage—for a few seconds or longer. If you're performing a crunch, you hold in your abs at the point of tension. TUT will increase strength, as your muscles have to work harder to hold the movement under tension.

Supersets are workouts where you alternate between two different types of exercises that work different areas with no rest between them. For example, you could do bicep curls followed by tricep dips with no rest in between. Supersets are exhausting in terms of cardio but because you're working slightly different muscles, they're getting to rest for a few seconds in between sets. Plus, supersets can be really time efficient if you are time poor.

Drop sets are where you lower the weight of an exercise you're doing once you've reached the point of fatigue, but you keep going with the exercise itself. Say you're doing crunches with a 10 lb. medicine ball—once you've reached fatigue, you ditch the medicine ball but keep doing the crunches.

Compound movements

Compound movements target multiple muscle groups at the same time and include squats, deadlifts and military presses. You need your workouts to incorporate compound movements as they're a great foundation for good posture, muscles and overall strength, which is what you want no matter how you organize your workouts. Once you've mastered form and technique, you'll find them pretty straightforward but totally exhausting.

MIXING IT UP

STRENGTH TRAINING IS my favorite but sometimes I like to add a little something different to the beginning, middle or end of my programs just for fun. I like a little something extra!

Plyometric training

Plyometric training is tough but a lot of fun. Think strength, speed and power—trust me, it's a lot more fun and intense than it sounds. Plyometric training, or "plyo" as it's known, encourages your body to build speed and strength in equal measure. It's about explosive action and speed, combined with power. A simple example of plyo training is box jumps, where you jump with both feet up onto a surface. That action combines speed with the explosive power you need to propel yourself onto that surface. A successful plyo session needs agility, focus, energy and coordination, so it's maybe not one to include if you're feeling tired, lethargic or it's a certain time of the month. Plyo training is used in almost every aspect of professional sports too. Think about those sprinters on the start line at the Olympics: plyo training is what gives them the explosive charge.

A good plyo session will work your entire body and combine cardio with strength. As it's such an intense workout, you need to make sure your form is correct before you start—that's why strength is important, as it helps build your form and posture.

Plyo can cause injury if done incorrectly; rest is vital. Where strength training is more about protracted movements and increasing loads, plyo is its little sister: quick, dynamic and exciting. If you're unsure about the movements, make sure you ask a qualified professional at the gym for guidance or modify the movements to suit you.

High-intensity interval training (HIIT)

HIIT is something we've all heard of and is about going flat out to the point of exhaustion for a very short period of time, followed by a brief period of recovery before starting again. It's been around since the eighties and nineties but has massively soared in popularity over the last decade or so. In our time-poor society, people are looking for a fast workout and HIIT can be as short as twenty minutes.

HIIT workouts are short because they're so physically demanding and draining. Although you'll save in terms of time, you most definitely won't in terms of intensity. However, if you struggle with explosive exercises, have a bad back or underlying injuries, HIIT isn't for you. Stay safe and stick to strengthening and correcting your form and injuries before turning to explosive workouts.

Steady state cardio

Cardio has long been one of the most well-known and popular types of exercise. From aerobics classes to zumba, aqua fit, running or cycling, all of us probably start our fitness journeys with cardio.

You know you're doing cardio if you're doing something that raises your heart and breathing rate and keeps it there while you work out. Cardio should be sustainable for a period of time—unlike HIIT. Cardio gets your blood pumping, which over the course of time improves the function of your heart and lungs. Cardio is mostly what school PE lessons are about (think cross-country running), which is why it tends to be the first thing we go back to when we want to make a health change. It's familiar, but it's not for everyone. I tried running years ago, before I joined the gym, and it's just not for me; I don't enjoy the monotony of it and I want variety in my workouts. My cardio workouts tend to involve steady skipping or changing up my skipping with mini challenges. Of course, everyone is different and if you love running, stick to it!

There are lots of different and varied ways you can mix things up and you'll find what's right for you as you progress on your journey. I have friends who love HIIT and some who absolutely hate it. There are days when all I want to do is compound movements and others when I quite enjoy a long uphill walk. Not all the principles will appeal to you at once, but they can be handy reference points for when you want to mix things up.

TASK: LIST YOUR STRENGTHS

We've discussed strength training a lot. Now I want you to write down your greatest strengths, when you feel your strongest and most confident. For example, I always make time for my friends, I'm always there to listen and I love that about myself. I'm always there for my community and I want them to know they can ask me anything and I'll always answer them honestly. I feel so strong and confident during my workout, especially mid-set! I love that feeling of getting stronger and stronger with every rep and I'm so proud of everything I'm achieving.

I want you to do more and be more of what makes you the best version of yourself—it's the best way to improve yourself and love yourself.

REST DAYS

WHILE I'M ALL for going hard with my training, my rest days are absolutely vital to me. There's so much you can do mentally and physically during a rest day. Where strength training is concerned, rest days let your muscles recover and build again, so they're as important for your progress as any day spent in the gym.

In the early days of any workout regime you may have a few aches and pains. If your routine one week comprises twenty push-up burpees and twenty bicycle crunches, expect a little tenderness until you're used to doing them. These exercises will all work dormant muscle groups you probably haven't asked anything of for years, so rest is essential. If you have continual aches and pains even once you're used to the exercises, take a few days' rest, then ask a friend to video you doing the exercises and compare yourself to what you see online. It could be your form is letting you down and causing some tenderness.

However, whether you're sore or not, rest days are absolutely vital because they let you do just that—rest. And not just physically, mentally too. The fortitude it takes to push yourself to finish a tough workout, the mental capacity and concentration it takes to make sure your form is correct as you increase your endurance, can be exhausting. Making sure you have a day off gives your body and mind the chance to recover. Don't forget, you're breaking down and rebuilding muscle, which is an exhaustive biological process. Your body needs glycogen to repair itself and get ready to go again. A rest day will help your body reboot and regenerate, so that your battery is fully charged when it's time to go again at the next session.

Rest days will also remind you of why you love the gym. If you go seven days a week, no matter who you are, you'll become fatigued both mentally and physically and it'll start to feel like a chore. You'll overtrain, put yourself at risk of injury, and mentally it will start to feel like a labor rather than something you enjoy. You should always rest to the extent that you can't wait to go back. Use your rest to boost morale and get excited about getting back in there.

Resting doesn't mean you don't have to move at all. My rest days always involve a nice long walk early in the morning. You need your body to recover, but like I said before, your mind needs a rest too. Use a nice walk outdoors to breathe and just be with yourself and your own thoughts—you'll feel so good for it.

Rest days can also be a chance to switch up your routine. I very, very rarely work out in the morning. I know for some people it's the best time of the day to smash it, but I wake up slowly and I hardly ever feel ready for a workout first thing. I always work out in the evening after I've finished my day and I like it that way. But when it comes to rest days, I get up early and I take Buttons, my gorgeous doggy, out for a long walk.

SLEEP

SLEEP IS ALSO a massive part of our growth and recovery. While we're asleep, we can experience a huge spike in the growth hormone somatotropin, which is responsible for recovery. So, rest in the form of sleep is essential.

Now, I like working out in the evening. I always block out a couple of hours: not just for my workout, but to take my pre-workout drink (see page 156), warm up, cool down, shower and get ready for dinner (see, like I've been saying throughout, it's all about scheduling). It works for my body and my body clock. Some people are morning larks and others are night owls. What do I mean by this? Some of us work at our best in the mornings (larks) and others perform at their best in the late evenings and night (owls). This also has something to do with our circadian rhythm. Your circadian rhythm is your body clock—your body has to do things within a twenty-four-hour period in order for you to function; sleep and waking up are among those functions.[4]

This can change throughout the course of our lives: for example, teenagers tend to function better later in the day (which is a bit crazy, seeing as school usually begins early in the morning!) and as we get older we may need less sleep and perhaps function better in the mornings. In any case, I think it can make such a big difference to your training regime if you can tune into your sleeping habits. If you can form healthy habits and design a routine that works around your sleeping habits, you're pretty much winning at life! I know it's not always possible (babies, high-pressured jobs, travel), but we can always try and so long as we build healthy habits, we'll always find time to fit in the right amount of sleep so we perform optimally during the day.

Some people say that if you train only a few hours before bed, you're bound to stay up and not get a good night's sleep; or, you should all train first thing in the morning to give you energy and set up your day. To some extent, the latter is probably a stronger argument, just because with the way our lives work now, training early in the morning means it's out of the way so we're likely to be consistent with it and it saves our evenings for family and friends. Plus, if you commute or have long days, you might really feel low on energy at the end of the day. However, it just doesn't work for me. My best ideas, my best performance, is always in the evenings. I come alive then! And that's not a bad thing, nor is it the "wrong" thing. I feel so tired in the mornings sometimes and I need my coffee, my book and a bit of "me time" to really wake up. Other people work in the opposite way and that is totally fine. You find a routine that works for you. Ultimately, if you are going to build healthy habits and this book is going to be your action plan, I can't tell you when to do certain things as that's not self-discipline. Self-discipline is recognizing your own lifestyle and preferences and understanding what routines and habits work best for you and your life.

After I train, I always get a good night's rest (or try to) so long as I have a good sleep routine in place:

- If I'm training late into the evening (after 5 pm), I'll tend to take my pre-workout drink (see page 156) earlier so that it is out of my system by the time I go to bed at around 10:30 pm (usually, unless I'm buzzing with ideas for work!).
- I use my cooldown and shower as my time to unwind. I try switching off so that my body feels completely relaxed for when I go to bed.
- I try not to use my phone or laptop just before bed (it's hard, but we need to keep trying to make it a habit) and I read instead of watching TV. Screens suppress the hormone melatonin, which we need in order to feel sleepy. You don't want to go to sleep wired as you'll just have a bad night, leading to a grumpy morning.
- I journal and write things down before bed. It's a great

way to get things out of your head (literally) and helps me feel more calm about the day or week ahead.

- I try not to eat too much just before bed, especially sugar. If I'm hungry, I'll snack on vegetables or have some water or herbal tea (non-caffeinated, like chamomile or ginger).

Rest and sleep are so important for recovery and for building strength. The two go hand in hand as you can't build a strong body when you feel and are exhausted. Eight hours of sleep is ideal. I know it's not always possible because of the lives we lead, but you should try to prioritize sleep as much as you can because it makes such a difference to your lifestyle.

CHAPTER 11

LOVE YOUR FOOD

Women have such a complex relationship with food. So many women I know—in fact, I think every woman I know (including me)—has been on a diet at some point. Maybe they've cut out a food group or only eaten at certain times of the day or increased their intake of something, believing it'll do them good, "cleanse them" or relieve bloating. The problem with diets is they again promise unsustainable results. They're too restrictive, they are dull and they almost make you fear food. Please don't be scared and don't give yourself a hard time about food. Trust me, I've been there and it's not good for you— it'll make you sad and frustrated and what is life if you can't enjoy what you eat? Most women I know love food, but we blame it for all sorts of things and give it way more power over us and our lives than it should actually have. We need to unlearn phrases like, "bad food," "cheat days" and "treats." We also need to unlearn that vegetables are "bland" and avocados are all you need to be healthy. Food is fuel, nourishment, colorful, tasty and what we need to be happy and healthy.

I don't really comment on the endless food trends I see on Instagram or in the news. Some people might think I should because of my position, influence and knowledge, but as I keep saying, you just have to focus on your journey. I want to train you to make your journey and your knowledge so strong and unwavering that you won't even think twice about the next fad that comes along. The way you do this with food is the same way you approach your workouts: keep it balanced, flexible, interesting, habitual and make sure it works for you.

If you're anything like me, you spend a large portion of your day (no pun intended) thinking about food. It's one of the biggest pleasures in my life. I wake up thinking about breakfast, move on to thinking about lunch as I finish with my oats, and by the time lunchtime is done, I'm already looking forward to dinner. I'm a girl who loves her food and it brings me a massive amount of happiness. As with everything else in my life, I'm grateful. I'm grateful I have the life, mindset and ability to eat well and I know my body respects me for it. Just like exercise, food is health and happiness for your body and you can build a healthy relationship with it too.

I grew up with mealtimes being among the most important times of the day. My parents are Albanian and, as in many European cultures, food was an important part of life. A reason to stop, take time, catch up and truly make a meal of it. It wasn't something microwaved and served in a rush— although I can be guilty of eating like that sometimes—it was a time we came together as a family. No matter how busy you are, food should be something you make an occasion of—that's not to say it should take you hours to prep or cook, it really doesn't have to. In fact, for the majority of us, cooking a meal usually takes between fifteen to twenty minutes, which is no time at all. Buying fresh and packing your fridge with plenty of fruit and vegetables means your meals can be varied and there is always food at home to eat. Here's the thing to remember though: you're in charge of food. It's most definitely not in charge of you.

I'm going to give you an overview of what you need to know in general, but I am a trainer, not a nutritionist. The knowledge below is to get you started. At Tone & Sculpt, we have a qualified nutritionist working on our recipe and meal creations to make sure we can provide tailor-made and personalized guidance for all of our clients. After you've read this chapter, go do some further research or ask a doctor about your particular dietary needs. Remember, always find what works best for you.

A BALANCED PLATE

A BALANCED PLATE IS made up of macronutrients and micronutrients. Macronutrients, also referred to as "macros," are the nutrients our bodies need in large quantities every day: carbohydrates, proteins and fats. Macronutrients are your calories, which are the energy you need to live, breathe and function. Micronutrients, on the other hand, are the vitamins and minerals we need in much smaller doses, like potassium, vitamin D, iron and folic acid. They're all needed in smaller quantities and have more specific jobs than macronutrients. Potassium, for example, helps heart rhythm and nerve function; vitamin D helps to protect our bone density and maintain strong teeth; iron helps transport oxygen through the body, which is vital when you're working out; and folic acid supports and builds DNA and promotes bone growth. Micronutrients are fascinating but, generally speaking, a balanced and healthy diet will get the majority of the micronutrients you need into your body.

You will see a lot of people counting their macros and calories on a daily basis. People do this for different reasons: to build muscle, to lose fat and for other health reasons (if you have diabetes or high cholesterol, for example). All of these reasons are absolutely valid and as long as you feel like you have a healthy relationship with food, counting your macros and calories isn't "a bad thing." It's become a bit of a controversial topic (we cover calories later in this chapter) because counting macros and calories might mean you have an unhealthy relationship with food. It can be dull and boring, it can become obsessive and, ultimately, it's not necessarily sustainable. If you're that person who won't go out for a meal with their friends because you're worried about your macros, or you feel after a big meal with family you're going to need to spend hours at the gym "working it off," you do not have a healthy relationship with food.

Counting macros is fine if it is part of a balanced and healthy lifestyle. You might say, "Hang on, Krissy, if I make it a healthy habit, then that's a good thing, right?" On the surface, yes it is, because you know what you're eating, you know your portions and you know what you want to achieve. But, if it becomes a habit whereby you don't enjoy a meal out, you get scared of eating certain foods in fear of going beyond your carb allowance or you just become addicted to tracking your calories, that's not healthy because you're no longer enjoying food as part of a healthy lifestyle. You're having to forgo time with friends and family, avoid food that you enjoy and, essentially, you're living in fear of food. We don't want that. All we need is knowledge, discipline and an understanding of what a balanced plate of nutrients looks like.

I'm not going to focus on calculating your macros in this book and there is a reason for this: I want this book to be about establishing a healthy lifestyle and forming healthy habits. I would rather you learn about how to treat food and understand that food is here to nourish you, rather than thinking you need to pull your calculator out and start eating in numbers. For now, this book is here to teach you the foundations of forming healthy habits, and an understanding of food as part of a healthy lifestyle is my focus for you. Here are some of the key nutrients you need to be aware of:

Our body's preferred source of energy, **carbohydrates,** gives the body the energy it needs to function day to day, but also to smash a workout. Carbs are broken down in the body into different types of sugar (glucose, fructose and galactose) and put to use immediately. Any unused energy is converted into glycogen and stored for when you need it—usually during your next training session. Carbohydrates can be found in pasta, bread and potatoes, as well as fruit, vegetables, grains and legumes, which also contain fiber, vitamins and minerals. These nutrients are essential to our digestion and other bodily functions. Eliminating carbs will result in a lack of these nutrients and probably make you pretty miserable and grumpy too, so do yourself a favor and learn to enjoy carbs!

However, like with fats (below), we need to be mindful of the types of carbs we consume. We love pizza and pasta, we all know this, but try avoiding eating too many processed and "beige" foods such as French fries and burgers. I'm not saying you should exclude them from your diet, I'm just saying you should keep your diet balanced with carbs that give you the right type of energy that you need to fuel your workouts. An excess amount of processed carbs can leave you feeling bloated, sleepy and dehydrated. Enjoy meals out with your friends and family—just approach it with balance.

Fat is not something you should shy away from but you need to know not all fats are created equally. Healthy fats provide great energy, support our cell growth, protect our organs and help with nutrient absorption. Good fats can be found in avocados, nuts, olive oil, nut butters, salmon, tuna, mackerel and dark chocolate. Unhealthy fats (namely saturated or trans fats), on the other hand, won't do you much good. You'll know what bad fats are, even if you've never really thought about it much. Think fried foods, cakes, pasties, processed meats, packaged foods and margarine. All the things you probably eat in moderation but know deep down they're not doing you that much good nutritionally.

Protein is treated like the holy grail of "fitness food." Found in meat, eggs, beans, fish, nuts, seeds, lentils and tofu, protein is essential for building muscle and a very important component of every meal. The reason why protein is so important is because it leaves you feeling satiated, it can prevent hunger and therefore it aids fat loss as you are less likely to top up with something sugary or calorific after a meal. For example, so many women think salads are what we need to be eating when trying to lose weight. If you want to lose fat, then you need to make sure there is an adequate amount of protein in that salad (think 1g of protein per pound of body weight) and that it's not drowning in dressing as, although it might be in your calorie range, the sugar in dressing along with the lack of nutrients will mean you feel hungry again in no time. You can even add some protein to your snacks, or snack on protein (beef or turkey jerky, chicken or protein bites) to curb hunger and leave you feeling full. Protein also has other functions in our body, including making enzymes, hormones, bones and even our skin cells. Protein is a "building block" and you need it—not to mention the fact it's delicious in almost every form—who doesn't love salmon or steak or lentils or cheese?

Fiber is a type of carbohydrate important for digestion and bowel movements. Present in fruit, vegetables, beans and whole grains, fiber allows our stools to pass easier and feeds the good bacteria in our gut. Another reason to embrace the carbs.

Vitamins and minerals play an important role in our bodies by helping to convert the carbohydrates, fats and proteins we consume into the energy we need. They also play major roles in wound healing, immune function and strong bones. There are so many vitamins and minerals and I can't cover them all here, so to give you an introduction, some vitamins to be aware of are listed in the following table.[1]

Vitamin	Great for	Found in	Anything else I should be aware of?
A (also known as retinol)	Eye health, immune function, healthy skin	Eggs, fish, carrots, pumpkin, sweet potatoes, leafy greens, mangoes, apricots, milk, cheese	Vitamin A should be limited in pregnancy—something to talk to your doctor about for more personalized advice Vitamin A is a fat-soluble vitamin*
D	Blood pressure; bone, teeth and muscle health; hormone production	Eggs, oily fish, red meat, sun exposure	We need it, especially in the winter as we don't get enough from sun exposure Vitamin D is a fat-soluble vitamin*
K	Blood clotting, wound healing	Green vegetables, milk, eggs, cabbage	Vitamin K is a fat-soluble vitamin*
E	Healthy skin and eyes, a strong immune system	Peanut butter, leafy vegetables, fortified foods, oils	Vitamin E is a fat-soluble vitamin*
B complex vitamins (B1, B2, B3, B5, B6, B7, B9, B12)	Protein synthesis, energy, forming red blood cells	Meat, egg yolks, nuts, leafy vegetables, lentils, fish, cheese	You will get most B complex vitamins from your food, however B12 is an important vitamin to monitor if you follow a vegan diet. You may need to supplement B complex vitamins are water-soluble vitamins*

Vitamin	Great for	Found in	Anything else I should be aware of?
C	Healthy skin, collagen creation, wound healing	Citrus fruits, potatoes, papayas	Vitamin C is a water-soluble vitamin*

*Water-soluble vitamins can be dissolved in water. This means they are easily absorbed by the tissues in our body. Any excess water-soluble vitamins we consume will be excreted through urination. Fat-soluble vitamins are dissolved in fat, which means they are absorbed better when consumed with a fat source such as oil. Unlike with water-soluble vitamins, when we consume excess fat-soluble vitamins, they are stored in our liver or fatty tissue for later use.

PUTTING IT ALL TOGETHER

P UT QUITE SIMPLY (and it can be simple), your meals should include a protein source, carbohydrate source, healthy fats and vegetables. Your ingredients should be easy to switch around: for example, you can make tacos with fish, vegetables or meat—the herbs, spices and salad can stay the same or be adjusted according to your palate. The taco is the vehicle and you can switch it up how you like. Similarly with stews, switch meats for veggies or vice versa; white rice for brown rice, you choose. Whatever you put on your plate, make sure it's balanced with different textures to vary each bite and keep you interested. Whatever you do, don't think every meal needs to be chicken, rice and broccoli—they taste good, but not for every meal—it is dull and unnecessary. Use this guide to help you make up a healthy plate:

Protein—a portion the size of your palm

Carbs—a portion the size of your fist

Fat—a portion the size of your thumb (could also be a drizzle of olive oil, for example)

The rest of your plate? All the **veggies**—eat the rainbow!

A healthy-eating plan incorporates all nutrients and includes the foods you love. If you are eating foods you don't like, you will never feel completely satisfied and eating will be a chore rather than a pleasure.

Supplements and deficiencies

If you have a wide, varied and balanced diet, with plenty of fruit and vegetables, you are unlikely to need supplements. Supplements are literally what they say on the bottle—they are there to supplement your diet *if* you are not getting an adequate amount of a particular vitamin or nutrient from your balanced plate. Some people take supplements because they are deficient in something; other people take a supplement because they want to improve how their body is functioning. Over time, supplements can help, but you shouldn't rely on them to be your diet's main source of nutrition. It's just not sustainable.

Pre-workout drinks are a type of supplement. They usually come in powder form, which you mix with water. Every pre-workout supplement has specific instructions to follow. These supplements have been specifically designed to help provide an added dose of energy for your workout. A pre-workout supplement can help if you're feeling particularly fatigued or you just want that added push. However, it is not a necessity and you can smash your workout without it. Some people drink a strong black coffee or eat a pre-workout snack, such as an apple with some peanut butter, or a banana and some yogurt. Just keep in mind that supplements aren't necessary and shouldn't replace any of your meals.

Remember, everyone is different, so it's important to consult your doctor if you do feel deficient in something. You may feel overly tired or weak, you may experience hair loss, acne, muscle pain or general weakness. You might even bruise easily. I always say that if something doesn't feel right to you, go see a doctor. They are the experts and will know best.

Deficiencies can occur if we eliminate food groups as this does not allow our bodies to function optimally. All the nutrients above are needed for our bodies—ditching one or restricting another just creates an imbalance that could affect your metabolism. Nothing is off-limits in my diet and yours should be the same.

Restricted diets

Just a small side note: if you follow a vegan or vegetarian diet, or one that does eliminate a certain type of food, this isn't a problem so long as you are getting the right amount of protein, carbs, fats, vitamins and minerals from the foods you are consuming. If you are going to try a vegan diet, you must make sure your diet still includes all of the vitamins, minerals and nutrients you need. It would be worth consulting a nutritionist or dietitian to make sure you make the right choices for a healthy lifestyle.

CALORIES

A CALORIE IS A unit used to measure energy. Specifically, the definition of a calorie is the energy needed to raise the temperature of 1 g of water by 1°C. All foods contain calories and plenty of women I know make a lot of their food choices based on them, but if we just focus on calorie counting without any context, it can lead to an unhealthy relationship with food.

A calorie is a unit, so it is as much a "thing" as an inch or a second. The term "empty calories" is often used to describe foods that contain calories but no nutritional value, so don't contribute anything to you in terms of nutrients. They might give you some energy but won't be as good for you as nutrient-dense foods, which will help with all sorts of bodily functions.

Empty calories are proof that not all calories are created equally. Foods like avocados are high in calories but they're packed with healthy fats, fiber and are nutritionally rich. A large serving of fries and an avocado contain roughly the same amount of calories but one is nutritionally poor and one is incredibly good for you. If you've ever compared like for like with calories, don't. Coke Zero may have no calories, carbs or sugar but it's nowhere near as good for you as water.

I'm not going to labor the point but if you've been the person that counts calories but ignores what those calories truly represent, you need to reassess.

Comparing the calories in a fast-food meal with the calories in a homemade roast is pointless because one is made from scratch and packed with nutrition and one isn't. You always want to opt for what's nutritious. Lots of my Tone & Sculpt familia tell me that fresh food is expensive. It is if you're not eating seasonally: trust me, I have noticed the cost of certain fruits or veggies soar once they're out of season! However, if you're eating with the seasons, fresh food isn't prohibitively expensive. If it's still out of your price range, frozen fruit and veggies pack the same nutritional punch as fresh ones, so if your purse won't stretch to fresh, head to the frozen aisle.

Whatever your budget, food should nourish every part of you—your hunger, your heart, your soul. Food is about love and you need to break any negative connections you've had with it in the past.

I approach eating with two mantras: if it's complicated, don't do it, and if it's unsustainable, don't bother. I can't tell you how important these two ideas are. If you look on the Tone & Sculpt app and see my recipes, they're simple, fast, fresh and healthy. What could be easier than a toasted bagel or some smoked salmon and scrambled eggs? The app does measure your macros and calories, but the food will taste so good and nourishing that your desire to count calories will soon disappear!

METABOLISM

WHEN I JOINED the gym that first time, I might have looked much like I do now in terms of dress size, but I wasn't healthy. I ate a lot of foods that were nutritionally poor—don't get me wrong, pizza still has a huge place in my heart (and very often my stomach), but back then I wasn't balancing pizza with foods packed with nutrients. When I was working long hours as a waitress and finishing my final law exams, food was what I used to keep me going, which involved a lot of fast food and quick on-the-go snacks, not necessarily things that helped with my concentration or energy levels. I'd eat late before I went to bed then survive on coffee until the following lunchtime. I had no idea what my metabolism was and I wasn't very kind to it, starving it at certain points then overloading it before I slept.

You might have heard of metabolism before, you might have tried to blame it for things in the past, including weight loss or weight gain, but don't give it power it doesn't have. Your metabolism helps to keep your body functioning; it helps you breathe, digest, and use your brain. All the natural processes that happen in your body that are second nature—the ones you don't think about—come from your metabolism. In order for your metabolism to function, it needs energy and pretty much all of your energy comes from the food you eat. Your body size, composition, age, gender and genetics can all affect the speed of your metabolism.[2] You can't really speed up or slow down your metabolism—it's not as simple as that.

Over time you can change your metabolism with strength training (the more muscle you have, the faster your metabolism works because muscles require more energy than fat cells do). But crash dieting, restricting certain food groups, binge eating and anything else that is not part of a healthy balanced diet will likely wreak havoc with your metabolism. Put it this way, if your metabolism is constantly battling with yo-yo dieting and does not know when its next nutritious meal is coming, it won't be kind to your body either.

This isn't me saying that intermittent fasting is necessarily "bad" for you. People fast for different reasons—cultural, religious or maybe medical. Intermittent fasting has seen a huge soar in popularity in recent years; if you decide to go down a particular dietary route, do your research and remember, we were not made to *starve*. Equally, as much as a balanced diet, weight maintenance and even gaining muscle has a lot to do with our caloric intake, I don't want you to become obsessed with calorie counting either.

There are so many different ways to manage your eating patterns. Dieting has become a huge marketing win for the health industry. Some people are convinced by a food philosophy that other people hate. The same goes for workouts: some people love spin, others couldn't think of anything worse! All you need to do is understand what you're putting into your body, understand what you need and enjoy a balance on every plate you create for yourself. Your metabolism will be happy and, as long as your workouts and food intake are balanced, your metabolism will work effectively for you. We're simple creatures and it really is as easy as energy in versus energy out.

A HEALTHY RELATIONSHIP

I HAVE FRIENDS WHO have one cookie, throw up their hands and then resign themselves to a week of eating junk food. Then they blame themselves, avoid at least one meal a day and go into beast mode at the gym because they think they need to undo or atone for what they've eaten. So many women have a negative emotional connection with food. When I started my fitness journey, I—like millions of women new to the world of strength training—thought I had to eat and train like I was entering some sort of competition all the time. I convinced myself anything that wasn't brown rice, chicken breast or broccoli wasn't good for me. I'd read they helped recovery and were packed with lean protein—so much so I stopped enjoying my mom's Albanian cooking. I thought broccoli and brown rice was what I was supposed to have, what I should fill up on. Don't get me wrong, it tasted okay and I mixed it up a bit but I stopped eating a lot of the foods that gave me joy. I had blinders on and didn't arm myself with the knowledge I needed to get a good balanced diet without depriving myself of anything.

Good and bad food

While food should be a simple transaction we should look at dispassionately, it's a feeling for so many of us. It's something that can cheer us up, something that can be so comforting at the end of a long day. For me, food is family, friendship and community. We have such an emotional connection with food that has to be acknowledged before we can start changing how we view it.

I don't want you to view food as something that's to be endured. Regardless of who you are or what your targets are, food is something you should love.

Food can't be "good" or "bad" unless *you* label it that way. Food is food and, my God, do I love my food. Give me bagels, give me vegetables, give me pasta, give me a glass of wine, give me chocolate. Give me all of it because I love it.

Yes, some foods might not agree with you and of course there are certain nutrient-dense foods you can eat to promote a healthy gut, healthy skin or to support you overall, but ultimately that doesn't make food good or bad. Too much broccoli would be "bad" if you didn't get your healthy fats and other sources of protein and carbs. Too much bread and pasta without a balanced plate isn't what you should be eating all the time either. My relationship with food now is similar to my fitness journey. It's taken a long time, but it is now a healthy, habitual and integrated part of my lifestyle.

Just remember, one salad won't be what makes you healthy and one chocolate bar won't make you unhealthy. It is what we do with each meal every day that makes the difference.

It's momentum, it's realizing that balance is the only way forward with food. The minute you tell me I can't have something, I guarantee I'll want it more, which is why I don't tell myself I can't have anything. What I want, I'll have, but in moderation. That's how I eat sustainably, without deprivation or restriction.

Just to add: if I were to give you a chocolate bar after you've brushed your teeth, would you eat it? Now, considering we usually brush our teeth first thing in the morning and before bed, would you eat chocolate for breakfast or just before you roll into bed? Okay, maybe at Easter, but you get where I'm going with this—the answer is no. I love chocolate as much as the next person, but I also know there is a wrong time for it. For example, breakfast should be filled with energy to set up your day and keep you going until lunchtime; a doughnut or even an oat milk flat white (my favorite coffee, just FYI), won't cut it. With that in mind, if you've been training hard at the gym, wanting to build a healthy habit, devouring takeout for dinner throughout the week is just going to create a barrier. Given the lack of nutrients in that food, you're going to feel tired, bloated and dehydrated—not the fuel you need to build healthy habits. Pizza, burgers, takeout, they're not cheat foods, they're not rewards, they're just food. Eat them, but don't kid yourself about what they contain. They're not "bad" and they definitely have a place in my diet but I know they're nowhere near as good for me as a huge serving of my fish tacos or my homemade Indian curry with a large side of seasonal vegetables.

It's no easy task because we all think about food emotionally—we celebrate birthdays and weddings with cake, we eat fast food on a Friday to celebrate the weekend. But they are all on occasion. The rest of the time you should be aiming to eat a balanced plate. A few squares of chocolate a day won't hurt—a whole slab, on the other hand…you get my drift.

Cheat days

If there's a phrase I hate when it comes to food, it's "cheat days." So many women I know have their Sunday as a "cheat day." I suggest you reframe the way you see food and forget the term "cheat day." Labeling anything like this will derail everything—there's no such thing as a cheat food or a cheat day, it's just food you enjoy.

Just by using that term you're subconsciously telling yourself that your regular diet is boring or not good enough and has no fun or excitement to it; that the foods you're eating the rest of the week somehow aren't enough or exciting—meaning you're less likely to sustain a balanced diet.

"Cheating" also implies something bad, which can in turn lead to guilt and the feeling that you've done something wrong when you've enjoyed a meal at your favorite restaurant or your favorite takeout on a Friday or Saturday night. You haven't cheated or done anything wrong; you're eating food you enjoy.

There's a growing body of research out there that suggests cheat meals and cheat days encourage binge and disordered eating. It makes sense as we're associating unhealthy and toxic feelings with food, which can create a downward spiral when it comes to food and our lifestyles. There are no cheat foods, there are just foods. There are no cheat days, just days. Suggesting otherwise implies you're rewarding yourself with bad food for the good things you've done. Banish the word from your vocabulary and do not associate it with any food or meal.

Remember, food is there to enjoy, so treat it like your wardrobe and your makeup; you want it to suit you, to look good and to make you feel good too!

There is no such thing as a "bad weekend"

Pizza, pasta, chocolate—they are all part of a balanced diet. For far too long so many women think eating out, having dessert or ordering a few takeouts means they've ruined everything and there is no return. It sends them back to square one where for some reason they feel like they've unlearned all the healthy habits they've built, routine goes out the window and they say, "Sorry Krissy, I'll start again next week."

Once you start, there is no stopping. Consistency is key and if we want our food and fitness habits to be ingrained and become part of a lifelong routine, we need to accept that all food is fuel and there is a place for it in our diets. We're not robots; you can train the human mind to enforce, follow and sustain healthy habits. We but we all have our likes and dislikes and we all have things we just can't resist.

For me it's pizza and chocolate. Put either in front of me and it will be gone in minutes. When I eat it, I don't feel guilty, I don't hate myself nor do I feel the need to run a 5k as soon as I'm done. That's not healthy and it will have a negative impact on your relationship with food. Instead, we need to be honest with ourselves and just be mindful of everything we eat.

A weekend of eating out does not put you back at square one. All of that food counts as food and toward your calorie intake—if you are counting macros or trying to eat more protein, so what if you had a great weekend enjoying the food you love with family and friends? That is totally normal! On Monday, you'll likely be at work, have meal prepped and have a workout planned too. You're always sticking to your routine—the most important thing is to just be mindful that, like with everything, you need to make sure you eat food in moderation too. If you were saying you have takeout every night or eat a giant-sized bar of chocolate every day, then we might need to have a chat about your nutrition. But if you're aware of what you're eating and you understand the balanced plate we discussed earlier, you'll also understand that there is no such thing as a bad weekend of food—we just have weekends. Some are extra lean, and others are extra sweet!

Ditch the scale

Weigh-ins should be banned. Well, that's what I think anyway. Unless it is medically advised or you're training for a bodybuilding competition, you do not need a scale in your house.

Scales tell you very little. There is a number that shows you what you weigh and if you're weighing yourself regularly, it tells you if you've "gained weight" or "lost weight." What it doesn't tell you is that some mornings we wake up more bloated than others. Some days our bodies retain water. Some days we might be a little dehydrated and on others…we might just be a little constipated! That number has messed with the minds of so many women for far too long and we need it to stop. In fact, I think that scales are guiltier than a "bad weekend" of food for why women stop training and caring about their lifestyles so much. It must be exhausting, mentally, to step on those things worried and wondering what the number will be today—especially without an explanation of what that number means.

Instead, get out of the habit of stepping on the scale and get into the habit of working out on a regular basis. Get into the habit of meal prepping. Get into the habit of drinking water. Get into the habit of being kind to yourself. If you want to measure progress visibly, progress pictures work much better and so do your clothes. Think about how you feel in them and what's changed. Stay in tune with your body too—the scale won't tell you about the persistent back pain that is slowly disappearing or that you can now run up and down the stairs without being out of breath. Those are the best markers—not the marker on a digital display.

TASK: CHECK YOUR MEAL PLAN

Get a weekly planner and write down what you will be eating for breakfast, lunch and dinner—and snacks! Look at it and ask yourself:

- Are my meals balanced (protein, fats, carbs, all the veggies!)?
- Am I looking forward to my meals?
- Have I varied and balanced my snacks across the week?
- Will I feel full and satiated?

HUNGER

PHYSIOLOGICALLY SPEAKING, WE'RE hardwired to want food. It is a basic impulse that keeps our species alive and is a chemically activated response that occurs in the body without us having to actively make it happen. There is a reason we salivate when we see or smell our favorite foods, and our tummies grumbling is a trigger for us to get up and go to the fridge. But it's how we respond to those hunger pangs and what foods we choose to eat that makes all the difference.

What if I told you that, although hunger originates in your stomach, it is your brain, in particular the hypothalamus, that is ultimately in charge of your quest for food? Would you believe me? Yep, it's your brain that tells you it's time to eat.

After we've spent some time digesting food from our last meal, our stomachs produce a hormone that our brains pick up on to tell us it's time for another meal.

The science behind hunger

Your hypothalamus regulates and controls your quest for food, after receiving hormone signals from around the body. These include ghrelin from your stomach, which signals when you're hungry, as well as leptin from your fatty tissue, which has the effect of depressing hunger when needed. Our digestive tracts produce ghrelin to tell us when it is time for another meal. But here's the thing: the stomach also releases ghrelin in *anticipation* of a meal. So if you've had a good lunch and you're not hungry at all, but there's an office birthday and the cakes and doughnuts come out, your stomach will start a feedback loop that will result in releasing stomach acids to digest the food it's anticipating you're about to eat. You're not hungry, you don't need that food but your body has produced a chemical response that is hard to ignore.

The thing about ghrelin is that your body produces excess after you've dieted. So when you restrict a food group or calories, your ghrelin production goes up, which is partly to blame for the difficulty of sustaining weight loss from dieting alone (especially yo-yo dieting).

Before you start thinking it's an uphill battle and that chemicals and their release can't be controlled, there are things you can do to lower the amount of ghrelin in your body.

Sleep is the best thing you can do to help regulate hunger. We're all told we need between seven and nine hours of sleep a night and research has found that those who get less than seven hours have increased ghrelin levels. This means they have more of the hunger hormone floating around than those who are properly rested. Also, if you go to bed early, you're less likely to snack throughout the night!

A 2016 study found exposure to **stress** increased ghrelin levels too,[3] so keeping your stress in check can help lower the amount of ghrelin in your system.

While our brain is responsible for how we *feel* about food, studies have found it can also be responsible for changing how we view fullness and, in turn, changing ghrelin levels. A US study split participants into two groups and gave them both the same milkshake; one group had theirs labeled with the word "indulgent" and the other had theirs labeled with the words "low calorie."[4] Those in the "indulgent" group had significantly lower ghrelin levels after they'd drunk the shake than those in the "low calorie" group. The "low calorie" group wanted more and, of course, felt they could have more as they'd just consumed a low-calorie milkshake.

Believing in your mind that you're not hungry could go some way to your body believing the same thing and reacting that way. In simple terms, we just need to be mindful when we eat—don't eat a whole bag of chips in front of the TV because, before you know it, they'll all be gone and you'll be thinking, "What next?" Don't think you need to eat the whole pizza because you've had a really stressful day at work and it will make you feel better. Mindful eating means you can eat everything you like in moderation and in control.

The science of the hunger hormones might not be something we can control too much but understanding it and realizing it exists might make you question next time whether you're really hungry or whether you're just tired, reacting to a stimulus or are just coping with higher than normal stress levels.

INTUITIVE EATING

I WANT YOU TO stop eating emotionally and start eating intuitively. I eat a bagel every single day. God, I love bagels. They're literally one of my all-time favorites. I love them toasted with almost anything on top. Just writing about them right now is making me want one (but I'm not hungry so ghrelin can do one!). I love chocolate brownies too. The more gooey and chocolatey the better. I love s'mores and popcorn and banana bread. Do I see them as cheats or things I shouldn't have in my diet? Hell no, because I also have plenty of greens and fruit and vegetables and grains and protein to balance them out.

Here's a truth you've probably heard: you can work your ass off in the gym; you can do reps and sets until you think your arms and legs will cave in. You can dedicate time, schedule it, form habits, set triggers, have discipline by the truckload and never ever miss a workout. You can do all the things we've talked about so far but if your diet is off kilter— if you're not putting the right types of sustenance into your body, the right type of fuel—you won't see the progress you want or have worked for in your mind or body.

Intuitive eating is a term you might have heard before but it's how we should all be eating—it's how we "used" to eat before the diet industry became the $33-billion-a-year juggernaut it is today. It's how previous generations ate before we became obsessed with measuring food. Intuitive eating is guilt free, and it doesn't involve anything being a "cheat" or being off-limits. It's making food choices based on what your body is telling you—and by that I mean tuning into your body and listening to what it needs as opposed to what you want.

You can pretend to yourself that your body is saying you *need* that stuffed-crust pizza delivery with ice cream on a Friday night—which is fine—but if you're always suffering with colds and coughs or if you're always lethargic, take a look at what you're eating and ask yourself if you're really getting the right amount of fruit, vegetables and nutrients your immune system needs to function properly. Intuitive eating is about making choices based on what your body really needs and what it tells you. It's about honoring the feeling that you're full and respecting the fact you're hungry. It's about stopping when you're sated rather than going back for more or finishing your plate because you've got food on it. It's mindful eating. It's proper nourishment.

Getting in tune with your body in the gym is exactly the same thing as being in tune with the food you eat and need. Focus on the balance on your plate, your forkfuls; go slow and listen to when you start to fill up. Eating intuitively is about listening to internal cues and getting in tune with your body.

There aren't any hard-and-fast rules about intuitive eating; it's not a diet. There aren't steps to follow but there are eight principles you'll need to stick to and, honestly, they're the most straightforward principles you'll ever read. Mindful eating and intuitive eating are similar—I'll be using both terms so you get a well-rounded understanding of creating and sustaining healthy eating habits for life.

1. Say goodbye to diets

The first thing you need to do is ditch the word "diet" from your vocabulary. Eating for health is not about starvation, deprivation or measurements. Healthy eating is not a diet; it's a change for life. We need to unlearn how we see diets: as limiting. From now on you are going to treat each plate with balance. This isn't about weight loss either, it's about changing your relationship with food for the rest of your life in the same way I want you to change your relationship with exercise. Yes, you may feel like you need to "lose weight," but as we highlighted in the chapter on strength training, a consistent approach to your fitness and food will lead to long-lasting, healthy results.

2. Nourish your body with good food

You don't have to spend a fortune on your weekly grocery shopping to eat well, but you need to invest in your health. Add the rainbow to your food basket: buy a range of fruit, veggies, meat, fish (or vegetarian alternatives, of which there are plenty of delicious options) and have fun cooking. Avoid microwave meals and too many processed foods (pasta sauces, frozen meals and fast food).

3. Food is fuel

Next, you need to make peace with food. Carbs are not your enemy. Sugar is not the devil. If you've tried diets where there are points for certain foods, forget about them. If you've tried plans where you're only allowed protein, get over the thought that protein is the only good thing for you. If you've eaten on certain days and fasted on others, forget it—every single day of the week is equal from now on. Food is here to nourish and fuel us, so enjoy it. Of course, if you have particular health concerns such as diabetes or high cholesterol there will be dietary measures you need to account for—consult a professional nutritionist and know that they will make sure you can still enjoy your food.

4. Get to know your hunger signals

Recognize when you're hungry and be mindful of your eating habits. When your colleague is munching away at their desk minutes after you've had your lunch, it does not mean you are hungry. Think about what you've had to eat in the last twenty-four hours; how many meals did you have and how many snacks? Did you feel hungry or low on energy before-hand? Did they satisfy you and leave you feeling energized? Recognizing your hunger cues and being mindful about how food makes you feel is very important when forming a healthy relationship with food.

5. Get to know when you're full

You also need to recognize when you're full and trust the sensation. That's easier said than done, I know. We're programmed to finish what's on our plates, but eating slowly and mindfully will let you pick up on the cues from your body that you're full or approaching fullness.

If it helps, you can pause mid-meal for a minute or two, put your knife and fork down, look at what you've eaten so far and ask yourself: *How full do I feel?* Really tune into your stomach and think about how much you've eaten and how much more you really need to feel sated.

6. Enjoy eating!

Eating shouldn't be something you do to get through the day or to get you onto the next task. Yes, eating will give you the energy you need to smash it at the gym or the focus you need to sustain a long meeting, but meals should be cherished and enjoyed. Try not to eat breakfast when you're on your way to the train station or as you rush out the door. Don't eat dinner mindlessly in front of the TV in the evening. Savor every mouthful and enjoy the experience of eating. Get out of the office for lunch, even for a few minutes, so you're not eating at your desk. Find pleasure in food and the eating experience. I want you to eat without guilt, just with enjoyment.

7. Take the emotion out of food

Emotional eating is something many of us do when we are stressed, anxious, feeling down or depressed. Why do we turn to food? Well, when we are feeling like this, we might feel empty, like something is missing. When we're stressed we're usually trying to fix something by doing "more." Food can help fill that invisible void and chocolate can release endorphins that make us happy too, which is why we turn to it.

If you usually eat when you're anxious or stressed, you need to work on finding something else to overcome that feeling inside you and get through those emotions. It could be the gym, talking to a friend or reading a book. But if you recognize yourself as the type of person who turns to food for emotional reasons you need to examine that notion and think about what you could put in place to limit the effect your emotions have on your diet. This will be a trial-and-error process—you're undoing decades of learned behavior—but it's worth it, I promise. Always speak to a professional if you are struggling—they are always there to help.

8. Hydrate, hydrate, hydrate

I also want you to eat every single meal with a large glass of water. There's a place for other drinks in your day for sure, but at mealtimes we want your internal organs—which are doing the work of digesting—to be hydrated and ready for action.

TASK: APPLY WHAT YOU'VE LEARNED

Follow the eight principles above with your next meal. Read them beforehand, really think about the food you're ingesting and make notes if it helps. This will ensure every meal you eat is designed to care for your body and health. Obviously, taking notes isn't mandatory, but if it helps you be more mindful, then give it a go.

Water helps break down food and allows it to move along the digestive tract. Water and the fiber within it helps with bowel movements; if our food passes smoothly, this helps avoid constipation and bloating. Our digestive enzymes need water to function properly, not to mention the fact that a glass of iced water is a thing of beauty. I love the taste of water. If you don't, try adding some chopped cucumber or strawberries to it. It's what we need to keep us going, so get used to enjoying it more.

Nutrient-packed foods will leave your body functioning well, restore your sleep and energy levels, and help your skin (our largest organ, by the way!). A healthy diet also decreases your risk of chronic diseases and improves your overall quality of life. Eating well and intuitively is awesome for your body and mind, inside and out.

In your new relationship with food and nutrition, your reward won't be the meal or the snack, it'll be feeling full of energy and health when you're seventy, because you've eaten foods that help maintain mental and physical health and keep you fighting fit for decades. You need to start seeing food for what it allows you to do and how long it'll help you live.

CHAPTER 12

DO THIS FOR YOU

The intention of this book isn't to give you a fitness challenge or a four-week transformation plan. It is aimed at your mindset, your thinking and your treatment of fitness, health and exercise. The final and most important key lesson to take away from it is that you are *doing this for you*. Every chapter, every piece of advice and knowledge I have shared with you has a recurring theme: fitness can work for you, you can do this and you will do this—and I promise you, you will love it.

Ultimately, I want self-accountability to be the strongest reason you stick to something, and while I have given you an action plan and tasks to start your fitness journey, there are several barriers that can get in the way of success.

You *meant* to get your workout done this morning, but a friend called, needing someone to vent to, and before you knew it, you were already running late and rushing out the door before you realized that window of time you were supposed to be sweating it out in had passed you by. Or, you *meant* to meditate this morning or work out, but the kids woke up early, they needed something last minute for school and your intention just fizzled out. Now, you're either too busy for the rest of the day or you've forgotten your gym gear in the rush to get them ready for school. Or, quite simply, you checked your emails, reacted and got carried away with work.

A common denominator here is that all of these barriers are visible—and you end up falling to the bottom of your own list. Children come first, a phone call distracts you, and checking your email first thing in the morning is quite simply the worst! I'm guilty of doing it too, but we have to keep fighting against these barriers. Like I've said before, strength training and healthy eating is meant to be challenging. Working through the challenges and enjoying the rewards is what makes it all worthwhile. You need to make your health, your fitness and *you* visible. You need to get used to the phrases "I need to," "I'm going to," "I want"—because *you* are important. *You* alone are your visible and tangible priority, *you* alone are your reason; a better and healthier and stronger you is your target and you have everything you need inside you already to make the changes you need. It's all about *you*.

You need boundaries. Boundaries are so important because they set the guidelines for how you want to be treated—in this instance, how you want to view and feel about your workout time and how you want others to treat it too. If the people you live with—your roommates or your family—see you prioritize the gym and working out just like you would a work call or seminar, those boundaries are set and they wouldn't dream of asking you to do anything else at the time you'd be working out. Equally, *you* need to respect that boundary too: switch off your phone and focus on the present. It is the best way to be time efficient. Boundaries help you prioritize and you need to get to a place where the gym and your fitness journey is your priority. Your gym time is your time. It's non-negotiable.

Commit to you

Everyone wants to be the fittest and healthiest version of themselves they can be, right? So why aren't gyms massively oversubscribed or the streets packed with runners and cyclists? Why are there countless specialists who deal with conditions that can be completely avoided by fitness, exercise and a healthy diet? One of the major reasons is that people don't take the commitment to their health seriously—they make a plan to be healthy but don't follow it through. They know they should move more, eat better, do more, but they just simply never seem to get around to it.

There are plenty of reasons why but often people think just the formation of the plan is enough; people assume it'll be easy to do because they've planned it. Like the first time I signed up to a gym. I thought the very act of signing up would be the motivation I needed, yet despite the fact I had a shiny new card and a letter coming to my house with details of classes, I still didn't go for two months.

Just planning to do something isn't enough. You need to show up. I sat on that gym membership for two months before I did anything, but if I'd gone to university or work in my tennis shoes and my workout gear, I guarantee I would have started earlier. I'd have started moving—even if I'd just tried one machine and been there for a few minutes I'd have started doing something. I'd have moved past the planning phase and into the action phase.

Take yourself and your journey seriously—commit, plan,

schedule and follow through—and you're far more likely to stick to it. Put your alarm on the other side of the room to avoid hitting the snooze button, dress like you're ready for the gym, make appointments with yourself, make fitness fun by trying new things and make meal prep a fun occasion with a variety of food! You can definitely do this and you will love what it does for you.

Every journey is unique

In the same way I'm asking you to adopt the discipline to train for "life" instead of just for a vacation, I want you to be disciplined enough to realize we're not all at the same point in our journey. Of course, I compared myself to other women when I first joined the gym but it's a pointless exercise. We are all different, we all want different things and have different lifestyles, bodies and minds. Train for you and only you.

Try everything

Even if you can't see yourself as the plyo queen, give it a go. It goes back to what I was saying about challenging yourself and living outside of your comfort zone. It'd be easy to opt for cardio because that's what we mostly know and it's better the devil you know, right? Wrong. Give everything a go that you possibly can. I never would have found strength training if it wasn't for joining the gym and being fascinated with that section of it. I guarantee you, what you *think* you might like and what you *actually* like are two different things. So whether it's spin, HIIT, weights or resistance, give everything a go and I don't mean just once either. Keep going back to whatever it is you're trying, at least a few times, because it's only when we know something pretty well that we can actually make a decision on whether it's right for us or not. You might have a frustrating first session of whatever it is you're trying but with a bit of perseverance you might start to like what it's doing for you outside the class or session—you might find yourself sleeping better, you're less out of breath carrying the shopping home or taking the dog out for a walk, or you might just feel a bit more comfortable in your own skin.

Whatever you try, give it at least two to four weeks before you decide for sure it's definitely not up your alley. Give every part of *you* a go too. You need to train every single muscle group with balance to make sure you're progressing and getting stronger in the right way. You cannot just focus on one area because everything is connected and your workout won't be as effective as you want it to be if you're all about your legs or your shoulders. You need everything to work together. For example, say you want to build your glutes but never work on your lower back and upper body strength. You'll find it really difficult to lift heavier weights, which will in turn pause progress and could leave you prone to injury. Everything is connected and working everything together over the course of a training program is how you'll progress and get better and stronger.

It's okay to have periods when you focus on one specific part of your body—a few weeks of abs or glutes or whatever you want that to be—but you have to make sure everything is progressing and developing at roughly the same time.

All your muscle groups are connected to something else so you need to work your whole body in order to be successful. It's the only way to be consistent and not get bored or overwork a muscle group and leave you prone to injury.

Keep it simple

Nothing will put you off an activity faster than confusion and not knowing what you're doing. If you're joining a gym, try not to overcomplicate your workout by looking at specific metrics or methods, like VO_2 Max or heart-rate training or intervals. At the start of your journey it should be as simple as showing up and giving something a go. Set yourself a challenge that you might try a new machine or piece of equipment for the final five minutes of your workout after every session; that way you'll slowly work your way around the gym bit by bit.

If you're going to your first gym session and don't know where to start, just section up the time you have there and move on after every five or ten minutes. Start with five minutes on the bike as a warm-up, move on to five minutes on the treadmill, then five minutes of stretching on the mats. Don't give yourself complicated distances to reach or miles per hour to achieve before you move on; instead, break your time into sections and keep things simple. You're supposed to be focusing on the exercise and how it makes you feel rather than trying to work out complicated algorithms about your heart rate, time and reps. In the early days, before those habits are hardwired, it can be easy to lose focus and energy with things if they're complicated, so don't make anything harder for yourself. Keep it simple, keep it easy and just focus on showing up and getting started.

Progress not perfection

This is easier said than done, but prioritize how well you're doing and how often you're doing it rather than achieving a "perfect" gym body—there is no such thing! If you're new to working out and getting your heart rate going, don't expect your form to be perfect or your reps to look beautiful. I've said it before, it takes practice, hard work and consistency. The gym isn't where you go to look graceful and effortless, the gym is where you are at your most vulnerable and your most powerful. It is where you finish strong and where you lie exhausted after your final rep or set. Each session is about progress, about getting better, pushing harder, doing more. It's not about perfection—there is no such thing. No one cares about how much you sweat, or how red you are. Your sweat is a sign of your progress so be proud of it. Keep a journal for a few weeks after you join and write down how you feel after every workout. Be honest with yourself and your thoughts and I guarantee you will start to see progress in how you feel.

In and out

I love the gym, I feel at home there, but I also have other stuff to do. Don't be fooled into thinking you need to spend hours and hours working out, whether that's at home or the gym. Remember, follow a plan, choose an amount of time you can commit to and just do it. Listen to your body: if it's painful, stop and move on to a stretch; if you need to rest, rest. Equally, if you finish early and have time for five-minute sprint intervals, do it! Don't scroll, don't respond to emails, just focus on you, your mind and your body.

Smile

If you're at the gym for the first time, try to embrace the new environment around you. Smile at your fellow gym-goers and within a few weeks or months you'll probably have made friends with people who are on a different part of their journey from you. You can either offer them advice or they can be the ones you turn to when you need a helping hand. You know that feeling of walking into a new gym or exercise class for the first time and how intimidating that can feel, so imagine how you would have felt if there had been a helpful smile from a fellow gym-goer.

Research has also found smiling during a workout can improve your performance—it's true! A small-scale study found people who smiled during a distance run performed better than those who ran with a straight face or those who frowned.[1] The mechanics of smiling reduce tension so in addition to being that welcoming face in the gym, a natural smile when you're working out could also improve your performance.

Approach your workouts with confidence and happiness— and a smile as you start and finish. Be proud of yourself and what you are achieving!

Ask for help

We all have to start somewhere. If you're going to a gym, make sure you sign up for the introduction session and don't be afraid to ask for help. Personal trainers are there to help and to answer your questions, and there's nothing we love more than that enthusiasm we see at the start of someone's amazing journey, so ask away and make sure you leave knowing everything you want to know. I remember the first time I walked into the gym to sign up. There were machines, weights, dumbbells, bars, mats—so much equipment, so much clanking and noise and so many people who seemed to know exactly what they were doing.

I remember my eyes darting around everything and everyone, watching what they were doing, how they were doing it. I remember wondering and guessing at which exercises worked which bits of the body. It seemed such an alien landscape; like everyone there spoke a language I didn't. But I asked for help and soon enough it was my landscape too. Don't feel afraid or daunted—it is a safe space, space to better yourself and be yourself.

TASK: SAY YOUR AFFIRMATIONS

I want you to take your time and read the affirmations below. I want you to say them every morning and know you are doing this for you. Affirmations, over time, can really help you feel better, more confident and empowered.

- I can do this.
- I'm strong and capable.
- I'm on my own journey and it will keep getting better.
- I will be the best version of myself.
- I will dig deep and finish strong.
- My workouts are my time to shine.
- I matter.

MAINTAINING PROGRESS

WHEN I FIRST started, I wanted a curvier figure, but I soon realized I wanted way more than an aesthetic change—my relationship with fitness has gone beyond how it can make me look. How it makes me feel is more important to me than inches on or off my waist.

This is your life journey—it's about sustaining your dedication over decades and it's about hardwiring those habits. While you'll get to a point where working out is second nature, you need to constantly check in with yourself. This comes from remembering your "why" and making sure that's always present. Set sustainable and achievable goals, be kind to yourself and remember your journey is your opportunity to do the very best for you.

Plan your workouts and food, use the Tone & Sculpt app or any fitness plan you like to help you. Just remember: it's all about building healthy habits—small steps will lead to big results. Your body is the best guide to tell you what you can do. Treat it with respect and remember that habits and routines are liberating; they give you power and flexibility to find time for yourself.

Keep the momentum going

A few times a month I ask myself two questions:

What do I want to improve on?
What do I want to strive for?

In my case, I constantly want to improve and perfect my technique, which will enable me to become stronger and better. I want to train hard, leave it all out there and know I'm better than I ever imagined possible. I have discipline so I want to be effective when I'm training. I also want to build more strength and become stronger when performing specific exercises. I want to beat the workout, not have the workout beat me. I want to be able to finish as strongly as I started, to roar at the end rather than whimper. I want my final burpee to be as strong as my first and, if I end with some skipping, I want to be as light on my feet as I was during the warm-up.

Momentum is a really important tool in continuing your workout when things get tough or when you get busy with work or your personal life. Momentum, discipline and habits are all linked: it's easier to form habits when you remember the momentum associated with your "why" and you keep asking yourself the questions above. It helps keep you disciplined and helps keep you going.

I find momentum changes with the seasons for a lot of women. In summer, when the nights are light and everyone's in shorts and T-shirts all day, it's easy to find the momentum to get to the gym and work out. The days seem longer and it feels like you can fit more in, not to mention the fact that everyone's in a good mood because of the weather—and everything seems possible when the sun is out.

When the nights start drawing in, I think subconsciously we all want to hunker down and be cozy. That's when the sofa can look more appealing than the gym after work. If you're reading this and thinking, *Yep, that's exactly how I feel*, you're not alone. However, there are lots of ways you can help yourself if your momentum is lacking:

TRY BOOKING A CLASS

If it's all you can do to turn up and you don't have the energy to devise your own routine, go to a fitness or gym class. You'll be told what to do, you won't have to think about it, you'll just follow the instructions and before you know it, your workout will be done. Whether it's spinning or zumba, you'll get moving and not have to do any thinking—and it will be a pretty intense workout too.

DOWNLOAD THE TONE & SCULPT APP

I know I'm biased but not only are there workouts and challenges on the Tone & Sculpt app, there's a whole community of supportive people who have your back and will encourage you when you need it. They've helped me more times than I care to remember and whether you need a kick in the butt or some sympathy, they're the best group of women I've ever found when it comes to support. The message boards are packed with useful tips and advice, and lots of women on there will have been in your shoes with whatever you're experiencing, so use that collective to help you with solutions, ideas, inspiration and momentum.

"PACK" THE GYM INTO YOUR DAY

Like with your supermarket shopping, errands or whatever it is you do on the way home from work, add your exercise and fitness into that. The likelihood of you going back out again to the gym once you get home is slim, so pack your gym gear, take it to work with you and stop by the gym on your way home. If you commute, the likelihood is that you pass by or close to a gym on your way home anyway, so make the most of it. Then, when your key goes into your front door, you know you're absolutely done for the day and you can plant your booty on the sofa without guilt.

TRY BOOKING AN EVENT OR COMPETITION

Nothing focuses the mind like knowing you have to go toe-to-toe with someone on a start line or in a competition. It's something concrete with a date set to work toward and, as we discussed, everyone loves a countdown. You're likely to have to pay to join the event and you're less likely not to turn up and waste the money. It'll keep your focus while you count down.

MINI CHALLENGES

Mini challenges can keep you motivated in a big way. Make sure they can be built into healthy habits and into your routine: skip for five minutes every morning; do ten push-ups before bed; take the stairs, not the elevator. Remember, not aesthetic goals, but practical, physical and achievable things you can build into your days. These don't have a time limit nor do they come to an "end," they just keep growing, developing and challenging you to be and do better.

TELL YOURSELF YOU'RE DOING GREAT

Take thirty minutes and sit with a cup of coffee or tea and really think about how far you've come. If you kept a journal at the beginning of your journey, why not read through those entries now? Journaling is a great tool to help you focus, to feel great about yourself and to keep you going in the right direction. Remember how hard things were at the start or how planking for a minute seemed impossible? Remind yourself of how incredible you are. Think about those times you've been on a streak when everything has gone well and you've aced it in the gym and remind yourself of just how fantastic those feelings are.

And that's truly what it's all about. Every transformation, every progress picture, every message—I read them all. I see how great fitness makes the Tone & Sculpt community feel and I feel it with them. What it does for you can truly seem unbelievable, but it is so, so real. I want all of you to take time, to be disciplined, to be consistent and just keep going. Just start. It takes one decision, one walk into the gym, one pair of tennis shoes. I promise you, you won't regret it; you'll love it and your body and mind will be so unbelievably grateful for it. It's all about you and it's all for you. Love yourself and get training! I'll see you in the gym!

FREQUENTLY ASKED QUESTIONS

I thought I'd use this space as an opportunity to answer as many as possible of the most common questions I get about fitness. I get thousands of questions on Instagram, Facebook and YouTube, so I've taken the ones I think you'll also be wanting to know the answers to. I try to address as many as I can on my social media channels, but sometimes having them all in one place can really help.

Q: Do I have to spend hours in the gym every day to get the body I want?

A: First, look back to Chapter 1, where I suggest that your "why" should not be based on how you look, it should be based on how fitness makes you feel. Second, no, you do not need to spend hours in the gym. We all have stuff to do and you can easily get an optimum and effective workout in thirty minutes. In fact, there are several research papers that suggest thirty minutes is all you need to get your muscles working, blood pumping and energy surging. I do not spend hours in the gym. I mainly strength-train four to five times a week and it is usually for around forty-five minutes to an hour, including my warm-up and cooldown. Depending on how I'm feeling, I might challenge myself to do another set or experiment with a new workout, but don't forget fitness is my career too, so when I'm training, I'm also thinking of how to create the best workouts for you! Forty-five minutes is ideal for a strength-training program but less than that is fine if you just prefer a HIIT or circuit-style training session.

If you're short on time, a fifteen-minute workout can be easily achieved too. We can all find a spare fifteen minutes in our day!

Q: Can I only strength train at the gym?

A: Don't get me wrong, I love training at the gym. I love training in a place that is solely dedicated to my workout, where I don't need to think about anything else, so I can leave the rest of the world outside and just focus on me. But I know that's not an option for everyone and it's not something everyone likes either. Your workout needs to suit you and you'll only train in an environment that is accessible and where you feel comfortable. For so many women, that is home. If you have kids, or you work from home, or there isn't a gym nearby, home workouts or working out in the park can be just as effective as training in the gym. People seem to think the gym is the only way to build strength. Let's get something straight, you can build strength in the park, at home, or pretty much anywhere with the right workout. You can get an effective workout in with bodyweight exercises, HIIT (see Chapter 10) and home equipment.

Bodyweight exercises and routines can definitely build strength; but, I will say that if you're looking to grow your muscles and build that booty (what so many people call "size") you need some weights. This might be a few sets of dumbbells at home, a kettle bell or even a barbell in your yard. Suspension trainers are really useful too—they are also known as the infamous TRX, which is an amazing piece of equipment. It's essentially a couple of straps that you can pretty much hang anywhere in your house (as long as it can take your body weight!) and challenges you to work against your body weight with gravity as your resistance. The exercises look simple, but they will leave you sweaty and strong! If you are setting up your home gym, I would invest in:

- Dumbbells
- Kettle bells
- A mat
- Resistance bands
- TRX
- A jump rope

You can build strength and stamina just as effectively at home, and more often than not, I find myself doing these workouts as life can get so busy. I feel strong and like I've won for the day every time I complete a home workout.

Q: Do I really need to train every day?

A: This depends on what you mean by "train." The CDC recommends we do 150 minutes of moderate exercise every week or 75 minutes of vigorous activity.[1] I tell my clients and my Tone & Sculpt community to choose a program between three and five days a week. Whether it's an intense session in the gym or a walk in the park, it all counts; it is movement and movement is so good for your health every day. Do you remember the section on NEAT (non-exercise activity thermogenesis) in Chapter 4? NEAT can count as daily movement too. But, don't think walking to the fridge to grab a snack or reaching for the remote is all you need to do. Think cleaning the house (I love cleaning), gardening, walking to the supermarket instead of driving, taking the stairs when you go shopping, the list can be endless and it can make you feel good about yourself. I'm not saying they're entirely accurate or necessary, but fitness trackers can motivate you to help with NEAT too—they can act as a trigger, the momentum you need to remind you to keep walking, to keep going.

Q: I want to start training, but I just don't know how.

A: Okay, so throughout this book, my aim has been to get you in the right mindset to "start." So if you now feel ready, revisit all of the tasks from the very beginning and plan your workouts into your calendar, take all the steps necessary to make sure you're ready, from packing your gym clothes and setting your alarm to getting your mat out. Decide whether you want to train at a gym or at home. If you are a complete beginner I would recommend following a fitness plan, like on the Tone & Sculpt app, or asking a personal trainer at the gym for some guidance. I say this because it really helps to have someone at the beginning of your journey to take you through a few workouts, to guide you through technique and form so you start to build confidence in what you're doing. Other than that, just start. Whether it is going for a short run, doing a home workout or starting a strength-training program, we all have to start somewhere and you can always ask for help.

Q: Can you lose fat *and* build muscle?

A: This is an interesting question and one I am asked time and time again. To lose body fat (what so many women refer to as their "weight"), you need to consume fewer calories than you are burning—you need to be in calorie deficit. But, by doing that, you're also not building muscle: to lose weight your body will use energy from your muscles to make up for the calorie deficit. Your muscles need energy from food to grow. It's just the way our bodies work—you need to be in a calorie deficit to lose weight but if you want to grow your muscles you need to consume more calories than you are burning or at least be meeting your daily output.

Although a pound of muscle obviously weighs the same as a pound of fat, muscle is more dense and takes up less room. That's why you'll notice that once you start weight training, you might weigh the same or more (although the scale is just a waste of space in your bathroom, in my humble opinion) but you feel stronger and leaner. So, the question is, can you lose weight while building muscle? The answer is yes if you follow the steps below:

1. **Eat more protein with every meal.** If you want to build muscle and lose fat, remember what we said about protein? Eat more of it and maybe reduce the amount of carbs in your meals. Your plate will still be balanced and you'll feel full as the protein will fill you up. When I'm looking to focus on reducing body fat and increasing lean muscle, I try increasing the portion of protein in my meals. So a little more meat, fish or tofu, whatever your choice of protein is.

2. **Opt for strength-training and HIIT workouts.** Try reducing the amount of steady state cardio you do and strength train around three times a week. If you want to do cardio, go for things like HIIT or an intense spin session. That way you are building muscle while burning fat too.

3. **Be patient.** Any kind of quick fix or extreme calorie deficit will mean you lose fat and muscle quickly, but you'll feel weak. And as soon as you consume those calories again, you'll start to yo-yo with your weight. Just stay consistent, do a decent amount of strength-based workouts and prioritize protein.

4. **Drink water.** More than 70 percent of our muscles are water. In order to perform well in the gym and to make sure we don't overeat, getting the right amount of water is key. Try to drink two to three liters of water a day—you'll feel more energized and more able to train too.

Ultimately, my answer to this question is to eat a healthy, balanced diet that prioritizes protein and to strength train three times a week or more. I tend to do five strength workouts a week and my favorite type of cardio is intense skipping sessions. Be consistent and you'll definitely feel strong and healthy!

Q: Is exercise bad for my skin?

A: I get this question a lot. I'm not sure where this idea has come from, but the answer is no. Exercise is actually good for your skin. Your skin is your largest organ and as your muscles strengthen and tone, they make your skin look great too. Plus, exercise gets your blood flowing, so with so much oxygen running through your body (blood carries oxygen to your cells), your skin will have a nice, healthy glow. The blood circulation can also promote collagen production and we all like that youthful, plumped-up look.

If you exercise without makeup and with clean skin, sweating can actually help unclog your pores and cleanse your skin. If you exercise with a full face of makeup and then sweat, this can lead to clogged pores, which leads to pimples and soreness. I get it though; if you exercise after work, you might forget to take off your makeup beforehand. I would make sure you cleanse your face thoroughly after the workout to prevent any flare-ups, but if you do start to notice your skin is suffering, then try your best to remove your makeup before you exercise.

You should also shower soon after a workout—staying in your sweaty workout clothes can cause skin irritability or chafing.

The other thing women worry about is stretch marks. Stretch marks are completely normal and yes they can occur as you exercise, from muscle growth and strength, but they can also occur from things like growth spurts, bodily changes and, of course, pregnancy. They are completely normal. Stretch marks are not bad for your skin and you need to learn to love your body. Stop caring so much about what you see in the mirror—there is no such thing as "perfect skin" and stretch marks are completely normal. They are nothing to fear or hate—embrace your body and everything it can do!

Q: How do I get rid of cellulite?

A: The answer to this is similar to my comments on stretch marks above. Cellulite is a build-up of fat underneath the skin and usually looks like dimples on your skin. We usually get it on our thighs, butts and around our stomachs and it is not harmful in the slightest. Again, it comes down to this image we have of "perfect skin" and a "perfect body." There is no such thing! The majority of women will have or develop cellulite and it is for a range of reasons: body composition, thickness of skin, age, lifestyle, genetics. You can't get rid of cellulite and there is no reason to focus on it either; you're better off focusing on training regularly and strengthening your muscles and bones. Yes, exercise and a healthy diet can help reduce the appearance of cellulite, but, seriously, don't focus on it. It's a waste of your headspace and your wallet: all of these creams, body brushing and treatments that promise to reduce or get rid of cellulite are not worth it and are unsustainable. Focus on embracing your body and enjoying your workout!

Q: When I skip or run, I leak. Why does this happen?

A: This is more common than it should be in women and it comes down to the lack of information out there about our pelvic floor muscles. Women think they only have to worry about their pelvic floor muscles if they give birth but it affects us all, whether we have children or not. Honestly, they should be teaching pelvic floor exercises to girls at school! If you experience leakage during exercise, it may be because your pelvic floor is a little weak and you need to do some pelvic floor exercises to strengthen it. Leaking happens to loads of women; it is most common after having a baby but can also happen just after your period or at random times. It can really put women off training and I completely understand why. It can be unpredictable, embarrassing, uncomfortable and just plain annoying, but it shouldn't be your normal.

Start performing your pelvic floor exercises (see page 33), also known as your Kegels, every day, even if you're not suffering from leakage. Prevention is the best cure after all. A few minutes a day is all you need and no one needs to know. I would always consult a doctor to help you with these if you're unsure about doing them correctly, or let your doctor point you in the right direction of someone who can help. If you are pregnant or have had a baby, a pre- and post-natal trainer can help too.

Q: I lost weight and now I have a flat butt and a flat chest. How do I grow my boobs and butt without putting the weight on?

A: Okay, so you haven't lost them, it's just that there are certain areas of our bodies that store excess fat and, for women, this can be our glutes, breasts, around our stomachs and also the tops of our arms. Unfortunately, we can't spot-reduce fat. What we can do, though, is train different parts of our bodies to help strengthen and tone muscles. It's really important to maintain a healthy diet, so look back at Chapter 11 (see page 147) to understand how to create a balanced and healthy plate. With this in mind, protein is your priority to stay lean, while making sure you're staying full and still working on building muscle. Don't cut out a food group, just keep maintaining a healthy plate.

The other thing to try is target-area workouts. On the Tone & Sculpt app, there are plenty of target-area workouts to show you how to activate your glutes, for example, and how to train different parts of your body to strengthen them. If you train consistently and maintain a balanced diet, you'll soon see the results you want. However, just remember, everybody is different, so this question is great if you want strength and stamina, but don't obsess over a particular image—just work with the body you were given. It's a gift, trust me.

Q: How do I get rid of hip dips?

A: Hip dips are not something to get rid of! I have no idea why this is even a thing. Hips dips look like your hips have been indented just down the side of your body by your glutes. I can't believe I'm even having to explain this as it really shouldn't be something that you worry about. It's literally just how your body is built—we are all different. It's like saying, "How do I get rid of my broad shoulders?" or "How do I make my legs longer?" Just stop!

But, it's not just hip dips, is it? We focus on:

- The thigh gap
- The double chin
- Bingo wings
- Muffin tops
- Cankles

These words need to be deleted from our vocabulary. Don't get me wrong, I've used them from time to time on myself too, and sometimes women don't mean to say these in a horrible way, they're just using a word or phrase that we all recognize. But it's wrong. It makes us look at our bodies in a negative way. The same goes for stretch marks and cellulite. Our bodies are different and the desired thigh gap really isn't a thing. Our bodies are all formed and constructed differently. We all store fat and build muscle differently. Do not focus on these mindless things that say nothing about how strong or awesome you are. Just stay consistent with your fitness and keep eating a balanced diet—nothing else matters. I'm not going to give this any more time or space and nor should you.

Q: If I run or do too much jumping, will I get saggy boobs or saggy skin?

A: In one simple answer, no. Wear a sports bra that fits you and the right leggings and tennis shoes, then your body, boobs and everything else will be absolutely fine! Obviously, remember, after having a baby or if you have a particular health or skin concern, your skin may change and stretch, but that doesn't make a difference to your strength or ability to perform to your best. If you do feel it is having an impact on how you feel or you find you are experiencing aches and pains that you shouldn't, it might be something more to do with your muscles and joints, which is when you should see a physiotherapist or chiropractor. Or, treat yourself and get a massage.

Q: Is coffee bad for you?

A: I love coffee! Coffee, pizza, exercise—my first loves. Coffee is not "bad" for you. No food is really "bad" for you, unless you have an allergy, intolerance or the doctor has said so. Obviously, caffeine is a stimulant and if you have several cups of coffee a day you might experience sleeplessness, a racing heart and even headaches. Remember, everything in moderation.

Q: Will protein powder help me grow more muscle?

A: Protein powder is a supplement that should be treated just like that—as a supplement. For a woman, the usual recommendation is around 40–60 g of protein a day (although this is just a recommendation). I give this range because different sources will tell you different things, and it depends on you and your body. However, if you're looking to grow muscle, the recommendation is 1 g of protein per pound of body weight. What happens if you eat "more protein" than you should for your body? Your body will simply excrete it or store it as fat. It comes back to the calories and macro argument. Ultimately, if you want to maintain your body weight, you eat a diet in line with that. If you're looking to build muscle, then you just need to ensure you are hitting your protein target, which nutritionists, some personal trainers and the Tone & Sculpt app can help with. But I want to emphasize: always, always focus on your health. Don't obsess over growing muscles or wanting to look a certain way. Be consistent with your fitness and nutrition, form healthy habits, be disciplined and you will feel your best!

Q: How do you stay motivated?

A: I feel like this is the whole book in one! But I get this question so much that it needs to be included here. There is no magic solution, I'm not some kind of superwoman, I am just like you. In fact, my community amazes me every single day with their commitments, their jobs, children, families, struggles, life challenges.... We all have stuff going on, but if you build the habits, discipline and, most important, if you prioritize yourself and take some time for self-love and self-care, you will find the momentum to keep going. Remember everything we've gone through in this book and, if it helps, go back and reread Chapter 1—you will find your "why," build healthy habits and stay consistent. Just commit.

Q: How do you run a business and still stay really fit and motivated?

A: This is probably my most asked question. I'm not going to lie to you, it is hard—and now that I have more than one business, it is *really* hard. But, like I said before, it has nothing to do with motivation. It has everything to do with my "why," healthy habits, consistency, discipline, balance and my awesome team and familia that surround me.

When I first started my Instagram account, I had no idea it would grow to the extent it has. I had no idea Tone & Sculpt would be a community of over 100,000 women and one of the most successful fitness apps in the world. I had no idea my vision and dream of wanting to make fitness accessible to all women would result in an app and now a clothing brand, which aims to cater to every single woman. But I had a dream, I had a vision and I used every single tip and piece of advice I have given you in this book to make it happen. It is all about healthy habits and discipline. There were (and are) days and weeks when I didn't get very much sleep or felt super-stressed, but my workout and exercise made me feel alive, happy and in control. It was my time to be my best and it then helped me do my best. I cannot emphasize that enough. How do I fit my workouts in and run a business? The same way you can too:

- I plan my week.
- My calendar and schedule are my life—literally everything is on there.
- I schedule my workouts and they are non-negotiable. Meetings and other commitments fit around them, or I make sure my workouts fit around my meetings. The two work hand in hand if you plan ahead.

- I meal prep and make sure I always have a full fridge.
- I always have a rest day, every week. It's when my best ideas come to me too, making me excited for my week ahead.
- When I need a break, I take a break. I am as disciplined with rest as I am with hard work.
- I limit scrolling and screen time; it's scheduled into my day like everything else.
- I practice gratitude—it helps keep me grounded.
- I surround myself with people who lift me up, who I love and trust—they keep me going.

My "why" now is to help and support as many women as possible across the world to feel and be better, to be their best—and that includes me too. That vision is strong and it means everything to me. If your "why" is strong enough, nothing will get in the way of the healthy habits you're building. If you find that you aren't able to be consistent or maintain your habits, readdress your "why" and find that belief within you to keep you going. Trust me, it's possible and I am living proof of it.

YOUR ACTION PLAN

Thank you for reading this book. I'm so pleased you've spent time—your time—reading it, processing it. Now you're in the best possible position to make fitness a habit, an integrated part of your lifestyle. I want you to be a lifelong part of the Tone & Sculpt familia, my familia, and I am here every step of the way to support you—I mean that.

I hope you've found the tasks along the way helpful. They have helped me since the beginning of my fitness journey and they still help me now; whenever I feel lost, confused or a little overwhelmed I revisit them. If I want to set myself a new challenge or try something new, I go back to the beginning and readdress my habits and routines too.

You are now ready to start. No excuses, no sitting back and saying, "I'll start next week." Start now. I'm here for you, but I'm also here to tell you that *you* have to take the first step. No more messing around—ultimately your health is your choice and you want it to be a good one. You want to enjoy life, your body and mind like you do your favorite restaurant—you always look forward to an excellent meal and you enjoy every last bite! Okay, I'm getting a bit carried away, but you know what I mean. You're going to finish this book with an action plan, a clear understanding and guide on everything you need to do to make fitness a solid part of your lifestyle. I want you to plan your next steps in fitness using the tasks in this book and the plan I've made for you here. Spend some time on it and really think about it—be honest with yourself and make sure you're transparent about your lifestyle and choices when it comes to fitness and training. It's the only way any routine or habit will last.

Every few months:

- Revisit your "whys" and revaluate how you feel about them. Remind yourself that you are doing this for you, to be the best version of yourself.

- Evaluate your fitness plan and how it's going. Do you need to change it up? Do you want to add in a different kind of training? Use the chapter on strength training (see page 123) to help you develop and structure your workout program so that you are always progressing and challenging yourself.

- Set yourself a new challenge—something to push you to new limits. It might be fitness related, or it might be something else: it could be mindfulness, learning a new skill or a new language—do something for you that challenges and improves you.

Every week:

- Plan out your meals and snacks and shop for groceries based on what you will be cooking. Remember to consider batch-cooking, freezing or online grocery shopping to make life easier.

- Set aside a portion of your weekend to meal prep and store meals in the fridge for the week.

- Plan your workouts and schedule them into your calendar. Use a fitness guide or ask your gym or a personal trainer to help you if you need guidance.

- Take progress pictures: remember what I said, it's not just about the aesthetics, the pictures mean so much more. They show you how far you've come and remind you of all the strength and power you're building on your journey.

Every day:

- Pack your gym gear or prepare your environment in a way that makes fitness easy and possible to fit in.

- Pack your meals and snacks for the day.

- Be grateful. Practice gratitude every day or as often as you can. Be grateful for everything you have achieved, every rep, every set, every workout. They all make a difference to you and you should be proud of everything you are achieving.

This plan will be something you revisit in a few months and I want you to come back to it proud of your achievements and how far you've come. Just remember: never stop learning, never stop wanting to be the best version of yourself and always remember your body and mind are capable of anything—you just need to believe in yourself and make a choice to start. Just start.

ACKNOWLEDGMENTS

When I was presented with the opportunity to write a book, I honestly hesitated. I've always been super expressive with the way I feel and I deeply value communication, but I really didn't know where to start or how to put into words what I wanted the world to read. This book could not have happened without the following two people: Jack Bullimore and Zahara Chowdhury. Both people play such a valuable part in my life and both understand my complex mind.

Jack, although things didn't plan out the way we may have envisioned, you have my unconditional love always. Remember when I first met you and I said, "I know we will achieve something big together"? You were driving me to work when I was a waitress and you looked at me and said, "'course we will." Although we have only just scratched the surface, I cannot wait to continue building something incredible with you. How insane it is knowing we started Tone & Sculpt at your mum's house and now we have the most incredible team with us every step of the way!

Zahara, I could never have written this book without your guidance, expertise and constant patience with me! I can't believe you started off by following my page on Instagram, purchasing my first ever workout program, becoming my client and now a dear friend I have so much love and respect for. You are truly a wonderful woman...a superwoman!

Writing a book is daunting but to know people want to read what I have to say is a huge compliment. Natalie, thank you so much to you and the amazing team at Octopus for all of your support on this journey. A book is so different to starting an app and it would not have been possible without your patience and support. Thank you for trusting me—working with you all has been a dream and I've loved every second.

Jenny, wonderful Jenny! Your voice and constant reassurance have meant the world! None of this would have been possible without your advice and guidance—I truly appreciate everything you have done. Thank you from the bottom of my heart.

Megan, you have believed in me since day one—literally! You have been incredible throughout and I truly, truly appreciate your support in everything! Thank you so much to you, Charlotte and your entire team. I love you so much.

To Sarah and Sacha, where do I even start with you two? Whenever I tell you I have an idea you never make me feel stupid, you never make me feel like I'm too out of my league or that I'm crazy! Well, perhaps a little crazy at times. You've always pushed me to do things I question myself on. You cheer me on and we have the best time doing everything together. It almost feels guilty working with you two sometimes because it never ever feels like work…it always feels like a new fun adventure!

I want to say a huge thank you to my mum and dad who taught me the valuable lesson of hard work and sacrifice. My mum worked three jobs a day to be able to provide a hot meal for us all and my dad risked it all to bring us to a land full of opportunities, leaving everything he had behind, to sacrifice it all to ensure we were better off. I may not say it enough, but without your constant dedication I wouldn't be where I am today. I love you both.

To Hollie, we unexpectedly met nearly ten years ago and instantly clicked, we quickly became best friends for life. When I had nowhere to live, you and your family took me in and gave me shelter. You stuck by my side when so many came and left, you had and still have the best intentions for me and my dreams. I can truly say you're a sister not a friend…you are my twin flame.

Finally, to the woman who could easily light up any room, make friends with anyone she met and gave so much comfort to a broken heart. My second mum, Nicole Warden. You saw something in me that not a lot of people saw, you believed in me more and more as each day went on and you never second-guessed any of my crazy ideas. I will never forget the day you let me into your home, while I was at one time "Hollie's Friend," I quickly became your second daughter and you my second mum.

I will never forget what you did for me, the home you gave me when I had nowhere to go, the food you supplied when I had no money to buy my own and the ongoing love you shared even though you owed me nothing. I knew that the minute I had made something of myself that I would repay you in any type of way. While you never expected anything I always wanted to give you everything. Buying you a dream car was one of the happiest days of my life because I saw your beautiful smile shine bright, you literally looked like a kid on Christmas Day, an image I will cherish for the rest of my life.

While the angels above took you from us sooner than we could ever have imagined, I still feel your warm smile and comforting heart around me all the time. While you may not be here in this world, you are always in my heart.

Mumma Bear 2, I love you unconditionally, I love you with so much purity and I love you forever and always. I hope to always make you proud x.

NOTES

All websites accessed September 2020.

Chapter 1

1. Sinek, S., *Start with Why: How Great Leaders Inspire Everyone to Take Action*, London: Penguin, 2011.
2. Godman, H., "Regular exercise changes the brain to improve memory, thinking skills," *Harvard Health Blog*, www.health.harvard.edu/blog/regular-exercise-changes-brain-improve-memory-thinking-skills-201404097110, 9 April 2014.

Chapter 2

1. Stone, P. R., Burgess, W., McIntyre, J., Gunn, A. J., Lear, C. A., Bennet, L., Mitchell, E. A., Thompson, J. M. D. & the Maternal Sleep in Pregnancy Research Group, the University of Auckland, "An investigation of fetal behavioural states during maternal sleep in healthy late gestation pregnancy: an observational study," *Journal of Physiology*, 2017, 595(24), 7441–7450.

Chapter 3

1. Elsworthy, E., "Average adult will spend 34 years of their life looking at screens, poll claims," *The Independent*, www.independent.co.uk/life-style/fashion/news/screen-time-average-lifetime-years-phone-laptop-tv-a9508751.html, 11 May 2020.

Chapter 4

1. Shammas, M. A., "Telomeres, lifestyle, cancer, and aging," *Current Opinion in Clinical Nutrition and Metabolic Care,* 2011, 14(1), 28–34.
2. Maltz, M., *Psycho-Cybernetics: Updated and Expanded*, New York: Perigee, 2015.
3. Lally, P., van Jaarsveld, C. H. M., Potts, H. W. W. & Wardle, J., "How are habits formed: Modelling habit formation in the real world," *European Journal of Social Psychology*, 2010, 40(6), 998–1009.
4. Duhigg, C., *The Power of Habit: Why We Do What We Do, and How to Change*, London: Random House Books, 2013.
5. Hammond, C., "Do we need to walk 10,000 steps a day?," *BBC Future*, www.bbc.com/future/article/20190723-10000-steps-a-day-the-right-amount, 29 July 2019.
6. **"Exercise and teenagers,"** University of Rochester Medical Center, Health Encyclopedia, www.urmc.rochester.edu/encyclo pedia/content.aspx?ContentTypeID=90&ContentID=P01602.
7. Shah, R. V., Murthy, V. L., Colangelo, L. A., et al., "The coronary artery risk development in young adults (CARDIA) study," *JAMA Internal Medicine*, 2016, 176(1), 87–95.

Chapter 7

1. Plante, T. G., Madden, M., Mann, S., Lee, G., Hardesty, A., Gable, N., Terry, A. & Kaplow, G., "Effects of perceived fitness level of exercise partner on intensity of exertion," *Journal of Social Sciences*, 6(1), 2010, 50–54.
2. Wing, R. R. & Jeffery, R. W., "Benefits of recruiting participants with friends and increasing social support for weight loss and maintenance," *Journal of Consulting and Clinical Psychology*, 1999, 67 (1), 132–138.
3. Feltz, D., Kerr, N. L. & Irwin, B., "Buddy up: The Kohler effect applied to health games," *Journal of Sport & Exercise Psychology*, 2011, 33(4), 506–526.
4. Plante, T. G., Coscarelli, L. & Ford, M., "Does exercising with another enhance the stress-reducing benefits of exercise?," *International Journal of Stress Management*, 2001, 8(3), 201–213.

Chapter 8

1. Hölzel, B. K., Carmody, J., Vangel, M., Congleton, C., Yerramsetti, S. M., Gard, T. & Lazar, S. W., "Mindfulness practice leads to increases in regional brain gray matter density," *Psychiatry Research*, 2011, 191(1), 36–43.

Chapter 9

1. Baumeister, R. F., Bratslavsky, E., Muraven, M. & Tice, D. M., "Ego depletion: is the active self a limited resource?," *Journal of Personality and Social Psychology*, 1998, 74(5), 1252–65.

Chapter 10

1. Quinn, E., "The benefits of lifting weights for women," *Verywell Fit*, www.verywellfit.com/why-woman-should-lift-weights-3119467, 2020.
2. Hunter, G. R., Brock, D. W., Byrne, N. M., Chandler-Laney, P., Del Coral, P. & Gower, B. A., "Exercise training prevents regain of visceral fat for 1 year following weight loss," *Obesity (Silver Spring)*, 2010, 18(4), 690–695.
3. Strickland, J. C. & Smith, M. A., "The anxiolytic effects of resistance exercise," *Frontiers in Psychology*, 2014, 5(753).
4. Suni, E., "Circadian Rhythm," www.sleepfoundation.org/articles/what-circadian-rhythm, 2020.

Chapter 11

1. Ramirez, N., "Women's vitamin and mineral guide," toneandsculpt.app/blogs/eat/women-s-vitamin-and-mineral-guide, 2020.
2. "How can I speed up my metabolism?," www.nhs.uk/live-well/healthy-weight/metabolism-and-weight-loss/.
3. Yousufzai, M. I. U. A., Harmatz, E. S., Shah, M., Malik, M. O., Goosens, K. A., "Ghrelin is a persistent biomarker for chronic stress exposure in adolescent rats and humans," *Translational Psychiatry*, 2018, 8(1):74.

1. Crum, A. J., Corbin, W. R., Brownell, K. D. & Salovey, P., "Mind over milkshakes: mindsets, not just nutrients, determine ghrelin response," *Health Psychology*, 2011, 30(4), 424–429.

Chapter 12

1. Brick, N. & Metcalfe, R., "A smile will improve your run, research finds," *The Conversation*, https://edition.cnn.com /2018/02/12/health/smile-running-energy-partner/index.html, 2018.

Frequently Asked Questions

1. "How much physical activity do adults need?" Centers for Disease Control and Prevention, https://www.cdc.gov/physical activity/basics/adults/index.htm. See also https://health.gov/sites /default/files/2019-09/Physical_Activity_Guidelines_2nd_edition .pdf#page=56.